Clinical Cases in
Physical Therapy

Clinical Cases in Physical Therapy

Mark A. Brimer, Ph.D., P.T.
Assistant Director
Department of Rehabilitative Services
Holmes Regional Medical Center
Melbourne, Florida

Michael L. Moran, Sc.D., P.T.
Assistant Professor of Physical Therapy
College Misericordia
Dallas, Pennsylvania

Foreword by

Charles D. Ciccone, Ph.D., P.T.
Associate Professor of Physical Therapy
Ithaca College
Ithaca, New York

Butterworth-Heinemann
Boston Oxford Melbourne Singapore Toronto Munich New Delhi Tokyo

Every effort has been made to ensure that the drug dosage schedules
within this text are accurate and conform to standards accepted at
time of publication. However, as treatment recommendations vary in
the light of continuing research and clinical experience, the reader is
advised to verify drug dosage schedules herein with information
found on product information sheets. This is especially true in cases
of new or infrequently used drugs.

Recognizing the importance of preserving what has been written,
Butterworth-Heinemann prints its books on acid-free paper whenever possible.

Library of Congress Cataloguing-in-Publication Data

Brimer, Mark A.
    Clinical cases in physical therapy / Mark A. Brimer, Michael L.
Moran.
        p.   cm.
    Includes bibliographical references and index.
    ISBN 0-7506-9637-0 (alk. paper) ✓
    1. Physical therapy—Case studies. I. Moran, Michael L.
II. Title.
    [DNLM. 1. Physical Therapy—case studies. WB 460 B857c 1995]
RM701.B738 1995
616.8'2—dc20
DNLM/DLC
for Library of Congress   95-13055
                                                               CIP

British Library Cataloguing-in-Publication Data

A catalogue record for this book is available from the British Library.

The publisher offers discounts on bulk orders of this book.
For information, please write:

Manager of Special Sales
Butterworth-Heinemann
313 Washington Street
Newton, MA 02158-1626

10 9 8 7 6 5 4 3 2 1

Printed in the United States of America

To Leslee, Jeanne, Eric, Christopher, Katie, and Michael, whose love, patience, and understanding made this contribution possible.

Contents

Contributing Authors

The authors would like to express their gratitude to a number of people who made this text possible. Practitioners who contributed cases to this text include:

Barbara R. Allen, P.T.
Adjunct Faculty, Physical Therapy, University of Central Florida, Orlando; In-patient Supervisor, Department of Rehabilitative Services, Holmes Regional Medical Center, Melbourne, Florida

Bradford J. Blanchard, P.T.
Physical Therapist, Springvale Physical Therapy, Inc., Springvale, Maine

Mark A. Brimer, Ph.D., P.T.
Assistant Director, Department of Rehabilitative Services, Holmes Regional Medical Center, Melbourne, Florida

Linda D. Crane, M.M.Sc., P.T., C.C.S.
Instructor, Division of Physical Therapy, Department of Orthopaedics & Rehabilitation, University of Miami School of Medicine; Staff Physical Therapist, Department of Physical Therapy, Jackson Memorial Hospital, Miami, Florida

Dianne V. Jewell, M.S., P.T., C.C.S.
Physical Therapist, Cardiopulmonary Advisor, Outpatient Services, Sheltering Arms Physical Rehabilitation Hospital, Richmond, Virginia

Edmund Kosmahl, P.T., Ed.D.
Associate Professor of Physical Therapy, University of Scranton; Physical Therapist, Visiting Nurse Association and Mercy Home Health/Mercy Hospice, Scranton, Pennsylvania

David Levine, Ph.D., P.T.
Assistant Professor of Physical Therapy, The University of Tennessee at Chattanooga

Emed M. Martin, M.Ed., R.P.T.
Pediatric Senior Physical Therapist, Department of
Rehabilitative Services, Holmes Regional Medical Center,
Melbourne, Florida

James B. McClure III, P.T., A.T.C.
Senior Physical Therapist, Department of Rehabilitative
Services, Holmes Regional Medical Center, Melbourne, Florida

Jeanne Moran, M.H.S., P.T.
Itinerant Physical Therapist, Northeast Educational
Intermediate Unit, Mayfield, Pennsylvania

Michael L. Moran, Sc.D., P.T.
Assistant Professor of Physical Therapy, College Misericordia,
Dallas, Pennsylvania

David G. Patrick, M.S., P.T., C.P.O.
Assistant Professor of Physical Therapy, College Misericordia,
Dallas, Pennsylvania

John P. Sanko, M.S., P.T.
Assistant Professor of Physical Therapy, University of Scranton,
Scranton, Pennsylvania

Gail H. Schuneman, M.S., P.T.
Rehabilitative Services Director, Department of Rehabilitative
Services, Holmes Regional Medical Center, Melbourne, Florida

Sheri P. Silfies, M.S., P.T.
Assistant Professor and Academic Coordinator of Clinical
Education, Physical Therapy Program, College Misericordia,
Dallas, Pennsylvania

Larry J. Tillman, Ph.D.
University of Chattanooga Foundation Professor and Acting
Head, Department of Physical Therapy, The University of
Tennessee at Chattanooga

Chris C. Wells, P.T., A.T.C.
Adjunct Instructor of Physical Therapy, University of
Pittsburgh; Team Leader of Cardiopulmonary Physical
Therapy, University of Pittsburgh Medical Center, Pittsburgh,
Pennsylvania

Foreword

Perhaps the best way to learn about any clinical discipline is to observe how practitioners react to unique clinical situations. *Clinical Cases in Physical Therapy* gives us an excellent opportunity to see how our colleagues manage certain patients under somewhat atypical circumstances. We are invited to watch over the shoulder of these clinicians as they carefully consider the best way to resolve each case. We are then encouraged to consider a course of action and see how our decision compares to the management used with each patient. Through this process, these cases lend terrific insight to physical therapy practice. We see how clinicians achieved some rather imaginative resolutions to complex problems. More importantly, we begin to get a sense of the strategies and procedures that will be effective in all our patients. By understanding what interventions work in the more extreme cases, we can better understand how these interventions can be successful throughout the scope of practice.

Clinical Cases in Physical Therapy embodies several other important aspects of physical therapy education and practice. All of the cases provide us with direct insight into the clinical decision-making process. We often see how therapists were able to look beyond the patient's primary problem or diagnosis and consider the complex interaction of factors that influence the complete well-being of the patient. Many cases, for instance, encourage the clinician to dig deeper to find the cause of the patient's problem rather than merely treating the symptoms of a certain condition. We also see that therapists must not overlook alternative explanations for a patient's problems. The most obvious reason may not be the real reason for a given symptom or behavior. Likewise, several cases remind us that we must not feel constrained to managing only the primary problem. We must consider other sequelae that can arise from a given pathology or impairment. These cases emphasize the fact that physical therapists are experts in recognizing and resolving many problems, and that we must use all our skills to achieve optimal results in each patient we see.

The cases presented in this book also characterize the emerging role of physical therapy in contemporary health care. We must consider and understand how physical therapy interacts with pharmacologic treatment and other interventions, especially in direct access and home-care settings. These cases provide us with a realistic and useful method for seeing how physical therapists can communicate with other health care disciplines to provide the most comprehensive care for each patient. The role of physical therapy as an integral part of an interdisciplinary team is reinforced continually throughout this book, and this reinforcement is done in an interesting and enjoyable fashion.

Finally, physical therapists often develop clinical expertise at the expense of some rather hard-earned lessons. *Clinical Cases in Physical Therapy* provides us with a way to benefit from the experiences of our colleagues without having to pay the price through our own clinical misadventures. There are many useful lessons to be learned through the decisions and strategies illustrated in these cases. This book will provide critical insights for physical therapy students and practitioners alike.

Clinical Cases in Physical Therapy is a valuable addition to our professional literature. These cases should be read and reread to remind us to think critically and thoroughly with every patient we encounter.

Charles D. Ciccone

Preface

The profession of physical therapy presents a number of unique patient care opportunities. Regardless of the patient care setting, seldom are there periods of time when acquiring additional patient care knowledge is not possible. This book is about what some ordinary therapists have done in some not-so-ordinary patient care situations. The cases in this text are unique patient care episodes that have occurred in the careers of physical therapists in a number of health care settings.

Many physical therapists have, at some point in their career, either witnessed or participated in a unique clinical case. In this text a *clinical case* is defined as a circumstance that required the therapist to analyze a patient care treatment situation in the clinical environment and work toward resolving an important patient care issue. The clinical cases presented in this book made a lasting impression on the health care careers of those involved. In many of these cases, the patient was "never the wiser" about what the therapist had done to assist in resolving the identified problem. The reactions and manner in which the therapist responded in a particular case cannot be considered the only approach to problem resolution. The responses and thought processes used by each therapist were, however, undoubtedly to the patient's benefit.

Not all clinical cases require a quick or immediate response on the part of the therapist. Some simply require the professional to investigate an approach to problem solving that has unique clinical relevance. Each of the cases do, however, reflect the importance of experience, good professional training, teamwork, and the value of wisdom and effective decision-making when presented with complex physiologic, pharmacologic, diagnostic, or therapeutic issues.

This book has been written for physical therapists in all patient care settings and for those who are completing their professional education. The cases do not present exhaustive detail and the resolutions provided cannot be considered the only approach to resolving the problems presented. The references provided at the end of each case presentation can, however, be used as a starting point for additional inquiry.

As health care continues to evolve, therapists will be called upon to evaluate increasingly complex patient care situations and respond in an appropriate manner. The cases in this book, although not everyday situations, demonstrate the need for approaching patient care situations from a conceptual vantage point. As you read each of these cases, make a mental note of how you would respond to the patient care circumstance presented. After analyzing the situation presented in a case, refer to the Resolution and Discussion that follow immediately. Ask whether you responded in a like manner. Would your response be more effective than the one presented? Your answers to these questions are important because the opportunity for you to participate in the next unique clinical case may be just around the corner.

Acknowledgments

College Misericordia physical therapy student participants:

Robyn Abbate, Melissa E. Ackerman, Paul J. Brower Jr., Michael DePrimo, Kristine M. Desmet, Douglas K. Fickes, Jeffrey C. Frail, Joseph J. Glazenski, Leslie M. Koscelnak, Michael Kurilla, Kristen Kwiatkowski, Nicole Marie Larner, Marlene M. Man, Lisa Nowak, Kerrie Ann Olexa, Justine Sperandeo, Robert C. Stahlnecker, Kimberly Stoddard, William R. Vitzakovitch.

1

The Case of the Difficult Staple

Today you are assigned to hydrotherapy to fill in for a therapist who had to attend an unscheduled mandatory meeting in another area of the hospital. The therapist indicates to you that your first patient has a full-thickness third-degree burn that involves the anterior compartment of the left lower extremity. The extremity also has a mild *Staphylococcus aureus* infection that seriously affects the ability of a recent surgical graft to heal. For you to fully irrigate the wound, the patient must lie semi-reclined in a full body whirlpool. Universal precautions and sterile technique are to be followed throughout the course of treatment.

The patient's physician requested you to be aggressive while cleaning the wound. In addition, to enhance wound healing, the physician wants you to gently remove staples that have new skin growing over them. In the process of cleaning the wound, you come across a staple near the surface of the skin that is particularly difficult to remove. As you remove the staple you suddenly notice blood pulsating from the leg while the extremity is under water.

What is your response?

RESOLUTION

Arterial bleeding near the surface of the skin is often easiest to control with direct pressure. In this case, the correct response is to leave the patient in the whirlpool. You may use the pressure of the water provided by the depth of the pool and direct pressure applied with a gauze bandage. By keeping the patient in the whirlpool and applying pressure to the wound, you allow others to make arrangements to transfer the patient to a stretcher if rapid transport is needed. In most instances, the wound stops bleeding, allowing you to gently irrigate the surrounding area and safely conclude the treatment session.

DISCUSSION

The preferred method to control severe bleeding is the application of direct pressure. In the absence of a compress, a gloved hand or fingers may be used but only until a compress pad can be applied. Blood clots should not be disturbed once they have formed. If blood soaks through the entire pad without clotting, the pad should not be removed; instead, additional thick layers of dressing should be added and direct hand pressure should be continued. If pressure firmly applied to the area does not assist in the control of bleeding, the extremity should be elevated and pressure also applied to the artery that supplies the involved area. In this instance direct pressure was applied to the site with gauze while the extremity remained in the whirlpool. The wound stopped bleeding within 2 minutes of pressure application without any harm to the patient.

REFERENCES

Michlovitz SL: *Thermal Agents in Rehabilitation*, second edition. Philadelphia: Davis, 1990.

Richard RL, Stanley MJ: *Burn Care and Rehabilitation Principles and Practice*. Philadelphia: Davis, 1994.

Shankowsky HA, Callioux LS, Tredget EE: North American survey of hydrotherapy in modern burn care. J Burn Care Rehabil 1994;15:143–146.

Thompson PD, Bowen ML, McDonald K, Smith DJ, Prasad JK: A survey of burn hydrotherapy in the United States. J Burn Care Rehabil 1990;11:151–155.

Walter PH: Burn wound care. AACN Clin Issues Crit Care Nurs 1993;4:378–387.

2

The Case of the Painful Calves

You are a home health physical therapist who has been requested to treat a 69-year-old man with a complicated medical history. The patient has a history of rheumatoid arthritis, diabetes, three heart attacks, congestive heart failure, and restrictive lung capacity that has reduced his vital capacity to approximately one-third that of normal for his age. Because of a recent and prolonged hospitalization, the patient is very weak. The physician has requested home physical therapy for assistance with gait training and activities of daily living. The patient takes a number of generic medications, including furosemide, ranitidine, sulindac, ipratropium, and diazepam. He reports he has been taking the medications as ordered.

When you visit the home for the first time you find the man sitting semireclined in a chair reporting considerable discomfort. He tells you he is short of breath and having increased pain during ambulation. He reports the only time he gets out of the chair is to go to the bathroom.

During the evaluation you find the patient appears to have swelling in both lower extremities with pitting edema. Both calves are tender to touch and skin temperature below the knees seems elevated. Manual muscle testing indicates the patient has 4/5 strength in both lower extremities. He indicates a willingness to try physical therapy but that putting his feet on the floor is too painful for him today. The patient apologetically asks if he could start physical therapy tomorrow because he is not feeling well.

What is your response?

RESOLUTION

After taking a history and performing an evaluation, the therapist decided not to initiate treatment. Instead, the therapist contacted the primary physician and reported the physical findings and symptoms. The physician requested that the patient return to the hospital. The patient was admitted with a diagnosis of thrombophlebitis in both lower extremities and congestive heart failure. In the emergency department, administration of dicumarol was started to assist in reducing blood viscosity. In addition, the prescribed levels of furosemide were increased, resulting in a body fluid loss of approximately 10 lb (4.54 kg) over the next 2 days. After 3 days of hospitalization, the patient was discharged home, where therapy was resumed.

DISCUSSION

Increasing demands are being placed on physical therapists working in the home health setting. Therapists not only have to be creative in the ability to provide care at home but also must be knowledgeable in the types of medicines patients are taking to assist in ruling out potential health care problems. In this case the patient was taking a number of medications to assist in breathing, to reduce anxiety, to treat arthritis, and to relieve an up-set stomach commonly associated with arthritis medication. The patient also was taking low doses of medication to reduce blood viscosity. Despite the forms of treatment provided, the multiple medical problems led to the development of thrombophlebitis.

The presence of thrombophlebitis can be identified by the presence of the Homan's sign or with a deep vein angiogram. To elicit the Homan's sign the patient is requested, with the knee in full extension, to dorsiflex the ankle. If thrombophlebitis is present, the patient will frequently complain of pain, especially to palpation. The skin may appear shiny and skin temperature may be elevated. If left untreated thrombophlebitis can lead to the development of pulmonary emboli and become life-threatening.

REFERENCES

Ciccone, CD: *Pharmacology in Rehabilitation*. Philadelphia: Davis, 1990.

Kloth LC, McCulloch JM, Feeder JA: *Wound Healing: Alternatives in Management*, second edition. Philadelphia: Davis, 1995.

Moore KL: *Clinically Oriented Anatomy*, third edition. Baltimore: Williams & Wilkins, 1992.

O'Sullivan S, Schmitz T: *Physical Rehabilitation: Assessment and Treatment*, third edition. Philadelphia: Davis, 1994.

3

The Case of the Athlete

You have been asked to instruct a patient at bedside in crutch ambulation before the patient is discharged from the hospital. The patient is a 17-year-old man who sustained a right tibial plateau fracture the night before while playing in a high school football game. There is also the possibility that he has sustained internal derangement to the right knee. The patient is known as a top college running back prospect who was informed by his physician that he will not be able to play for the rest of the season.

While you are reading the patient's chart before going to his room, a worker on the orthopedic floor indicates that the athlete made continual requests for pain medication during the night and has been very difficult for the staff to manage. The patient is reported to be angry over his situation and does not want to be bothered. His physician has not seen him since applying a full leg cast in the emergency department the night before your visit.

Upon evaluation, you find the patient appears to be in pain and refuses to attempt ambulation. His leg has been elevated on two pillows with an ice pack applied to the site of the fracture. The foot is swollen, and the patient reports numbness over the dorsum of the foot. You ask the patient to flex and extend his toes. He responds by flexing the toes but extension cannot be seen or palpated. The patient abruptly responds, "I've had enough. Please just leave me alone!"

How would you respond?

RESOLUTION

The therapist in this situation examined the cast to see if it had been fitted too tightly. Because the patient had a full leg cast, an attempt was made to palpate the area around the toes on the dorsal and plantar surfaces of the foot. Noting that the space was minimal at best, the therapist asked that the physician be contacted regarding the possibility that the cast was too tight. The physician immediately ordered the cast be windowed laterally to relieve pressure from the peroneal nerve over the head of the fibula. Within 30 minutes the numbness on the dorsum of the patient's foot had largely cleared, and the patient was able to partially extend his toes. The patient received a new cast and experienced no additional difficulties.

DISCUSSION

Had reducing the pressure not been effective and loss of motor function remained, the physician would have been faced with the possibility of treating an anterior compartment syndrome. A compartment syndrome can occur within a muscle-group compartment in either the upper or lower extremity as a result of a severe blow to the muscle group involved. Pressure due to internal bleeding and swelling can, in severe traumatic conditions, compromise blood circulation to the involved area. Prolonged pressure and lack of circulation within a compartment may cause tissue to become gangrenous, necessitating surgical intervention.

The onset of a compartment syndrome, if it is going to occur, is usually quite rapid after severe trauma. As time passes, the likelihood of development decreases. To relieve the pressure associated with anterior compartment syndrome, the physician must quickly perform surgical fasciotomy of the anterior compartment to prevent long-term nerve or muscle damage.

REFERENCES

Andrews JR, Teddler JL, Godbout BP: Bicondylar tibial plateau fracture complicated by compartment syndrome. Orthop Rev 1992;21:317–319.

Kaeser HE: Polyneuropathies with a abnormal tendency for pressure-induced paralysis. Schweiz Rundsch Med Pract 1992;81:1250–1253.

Magee DJ: *Orthopedic Physical Therapy*, second edition. Philadelphia: Saunders, 1992.

4

The Case of the Basketball Player

A 23-year-old man has been referred to your facility for physical therapy after sustaining an injury to the right knee while playing intramural basketball 1 week ago. The patient was initially evaluated in the emergency department and referred to an orthopedic surgeon. The patient was seen once in the office of an orthopedic surgeon who aspirated about 20 mL of blood from the knee.

The injury was sustained when the patient was rebounding and felt the knee give way when he came down with the ball. The physician suspects the terrible triad—injury to the medial collateral ligament, medial meniscus, and the anterior cruciate ligament. The patient wants to attempt physical therapy for a period of time before agreeing to arthroscopic surgery or any form of reconstruction.

Upon evaluation, you find the patient bearing partial weight on the leg with the use of crutches. The knee is very warm and sensitive to light touch, and range of motion is painful with flexion to only 70 degrees and extension limited to –15 degrees. The patient indicates he has been running a low-grade fever of 99 degrees and reports that he generally has not been feeling well. The physician has prescribed a nonsteroidal anti-inflammatory drug and asked the patient to return to the office in 1 week. The physician has requested a physical therapist to initiate range of motion and progress weight-bearing as tolerated. The first treatment session (consisting of gentle range of motion) does not go well because the patient experiences severe pain and makes no discernible progress in obtaining any additional range of motion.

What potential problem do you suspect?

RESOLUTION

The therapist in this instance recognized the problem as possibly related to an infection in the knee joint. The physician's office was immediately contacted and apprised of the symptoms. The patient was seen by the physician later that same day and subsequently admitted to the hospital. The next day the patient underwent arthroscopic surgery and was given intravenous antibiotics for 7 days. The patient apparently had contracted a staphylococcal infection of the knee during aspiration of the joint. Once the infection was under control, the patient resumed physical therapy.

DISCUSSION

Higher levels of education have added increased responsibility to the profession of physical therapy. Therapists must recognize when a patient is experiencing unusual difficulty and be willing to intercede when problems arise. This is particularly important when the patient is not scheduled for follow-up with the physician for an extended period of time.

REFERENCES

Barber FA: What is the terrible triad? Arthroscopy 1992;8:19–22.

Neinstein LS: *Adolescent Health Care: A Practical Guide*, second edition. Baltimore: Williams & Wilkins, 1991.

Shannon MT, Wilson BA: *Govoni & Hayes: Drugs and Nursing Implications*, seventh edition. East Norwalk: Appleton & Lange, 1992.

Walter JB: *An Introduction to the Principles of Disease*, third edition. Philadelphia: Saunders, 1992.

5

The Case of Eye Contamination

You are one of two therapists assigned to work in the hydrotherapy department of a 250-bed acute care hospital. For the
past 2 weeks you have been treating in hydrotherapy a very ill
HIV-positive patient who has open wounds. A large portion of
the area you are debriding is very painful and frequently
bleeds into the whirlpool.

The patient generally tolerates wound debridement. Today,
however, as you are cleaning the wound the patient suddenly
moves because of pain. The sudden movement, completely accidental, splashes water into the other therapist's face and directly into her eye. The therapist immediately drops her
debridement tools and jumps back, requesting that someone
provide her with a towel.

How would you respond in this situation?

RESOLUTION

The first therapist calmed the patient and quickly came to the assistance of the therapist who had been splashed with the contaminated water. She helped wipe the therapist's face and then used an eye irrigation system available within the department to cleanse and irrigate the eye. Although no water had gone into the mouth, the first therapist rinsed the splashed therapist's mouth with 10% by volume hydrogen peroxide. The splashed therapist was taken to the emergency department, where the eye was irrigated again and blood samples were taken to establish a baseline with which to monitor exposure to the HIV virus. The accident was documented with an incident report. To date, additional tests have been negative for the presence of HIV.

Since the splash incident, departmental policies and procedures have been changed. The entire department has been instructed in the proper mechanisms to use in the event of a similar incident. Anyone working in the hydrotherapy department must now wear a face shield to prevent another event such as the one described.

DISCUSSION

Although there are no documented instances of a health care worker's contracting HIV through hydrotherapy, exposure safety precautions must be followed. Besides wearing proper clothing, it is important to add chemical disinfectants to the water to lessen the probability of exposure should a splash occur. In this instance the water had been treated with chemical disinfectants before the initiation of debridement.

REFERENCES

Kloth LC, McCulloch JM, Feeder JA: *Wound Healing: Alternatives in Management*, second edition. Philadelphia: Davis, 1995.

Lynch P, Cummings J, Robert PL, Heuriott MJ, Yates B, Stamm WE: Implementing and evaluating a system of generic infection precautions: body substance isolation. Am J Infect Control 1990;18:1.

Oakley K: Making sense of accidental exposure to blood and body fluids. Nurs Times 1992;88:40–42.

Occupational Safety and Health Administration's Blood Borne Pathogen Reference Guide. Department of Labor Federal Register. December 6, 1991, Vol 56.

Sheehy SB, Marvin JA, Jimmerson CL: *Manual of Clinical Trauma Care: The First Hour.* St. Louis: Mosby, 1989.

Universal Blood and Body Substance Precautions: Specific Guidelines, sixth edition. Wichita: APIC, 1992.

6

The Case of the Painful Neck

You have been requested by one of the therapists who works in your department to assist in the reassessment of a 44-year-old woman who is recovering from a whiplash injury as a result of an automobile accident. The accident occurred 1 month ago. The patient was a passenger in a stationary vehicle that was struck from behind by another automobile traveling approximately 30 miles per hour. She has been out of work and at home taking prescribed medication. Her physician had requested the patient receive moist heat, cervical traction, gentle range of motion, and a home program.

Therapy provided for the past 2 weeks has made little progress in alleviating the patient's symptoms. After receiving therapy, the patient indicates that she often feels worse. After some of the treatment sessions she complains of dizziness and nausea. The patient is clearly becoming frustrated, and the therapist is concerned that application of heat may be a source of the problem.

Upon evaluation, you find the patient very apprehensive and reporting considerable neck pain. The trapezius muscle has marked bilateral spasm and is tender to palpation. Sensation is intact in the upper extremities. Both upper extremities present full range of motion. To ascertain the patient's range of motion in the cervical spine you request that she lie supine while you support her head. During the evaluation of cervical range of motion you attempt to rotate her head while holding the cervical spine in an extended position. In the process of slowly rotating her head, you note slight nystagmus. The patient immediately reports dizziness and nausea.

What problem do you suspect?

RESOLUTION

By performing the motion described, the therapist evaluates the integrity of the circulation provided by the vertebral artery. The vertebral artery test is considered positive if the patient presents symptoms of nystagmus, altered pupil dilatation, or slurred speech. A positive test indicates the patient may not have sufficient collateral circulation if the vertebral artery is compromised. For an adequate test, the patient lies supine and the therapist holds the head with the neck rotated and extended for 15 seconds. There should be a 30-second rest in the neutral position before range of motion is tested in the opposite direction. Patients are instructed to keep their eyes open during the test. Patients with vertebral artery problems often report dizziness, ringing in the ears, nausea, or blurred vision when the test is performed.

DISCUSSION

When a patient has a positive vertebral artery test, motions and treatment regimens that include a combination of cervical extension and rotation should be avoided. Prolonged compromise of collateral circulation may be harmful. In this case the therapist developed a plan of care that did not include the application of cervical traction. Instead the therapist applied moist heat and ultrasound and used a stretching program that helped address spasm in the upper trapezius. The patient underwent therapy for 1 month and was discharged to a home program of stretching and strengthening. The home program was designed to follow up the care she received at the facility.

REFERENCES

Hecox B, Mehreteab TA, Weisberg J: *Physical Agents.* East Norwalk: Appleton & Lange, 1994.

Magee DJ: *Orthopedic Physical Assessment,* second edition. Philadelphia: Saunders, 1992.

Richardson JK, Iglarsh ZA: *Clinical Orthopedic Physical Therapy.* Philadelphia: Saunders, 1994.

7

The Case of the Computer Engineer

A 26-year-old computer engineer arrives at your clinic for evaluation and treatment. The woman is employed at a research center that designs some of the latest computer software for military aircraft. The job she has is demanding and requires many long hours of professional dedication.

Over the past 2 months the job seems to have taken its physical toll on the patient. Among other symptoms, she reports fatigue at the end of each day and has difficulty maintaining her energy level. Because the patient spends many long hours seated in front of a computer terminal, her physician has requested her to begin exercise on a regular basis but in a manner supervised and under the direction of a physical therapist. As her therapist, one of your primary goals is to make sure the patient follows a specifically prescribed program in the initial stages. Once you have her off to a good start, the objective is to have her continue the program you have designed at a local fitness center.

After 3 weeks of therapy that emphasized progressive therapeutic exercise, the patient seems to be making little progress in general conditioning. She reports fatigue, general lack of energy, weight loss, and that generalized muscle aches and joint pains are unchanged even though she has made great strides in cutting back on hours spent at work. She also reports visual difficulties with one eye and feels as though she is dragging one of her legs. She is becoming frustrated and discouraged and is ready to give up on therapy.

What would you recommend be done next?

RESOLUTION

The therapist recognized the lack of progress and apparent deterioration in visual acuity as symptoms of a larger problem. The therapist contacted the referring physician and inquired about any history of neurologic illness. After the therapist discussed the clinical findings and their relevance, the physician immediately referred the patient to a neurologist. Upon evaluation the neurologist provided a tentative diagnosis of multiple sclerosis, which necessitated a change in physical therapy. The new plan of care was one that emphasized environmental and lifestyle modifications to help compensate for the movement dysfunctions commonly associated with multiple sclerosis.

DISCUSSION

The diagnosis of multiple sclerosis may be difficult in the early stages of the illness. Some of the classic features of the disease include motor weakness, paresthesia, diplopia, nystagmus, dysarthria, ataxia, impairment of deep sensation, and alteration of emotional responses. In some instances 1 to 10 years may elapse between the initial symptom and subsequent symptoms that help in obtaining a definitive diagnosis. As a rule, the diagnosis of multiple sclerosis cannot be certain until there is a history of remission and relapse and evidence of central nervous system involvement.

REFERENCES

Adams R, Victor M: *Principles of Neurology,* third edition. New York: McGraw-Hill, 1985.

Frankel D: *Neurological Rehabilitation,* second edition. St. Louis: Mosby, 1990.

Hoffman M: On the trail of the errant T cells of multiple sclerosis. Science 1991;254:521.

Kandel E, Schwartz JT: *Principles of Neural Science,* third edition. New York: Elsevier, 1991.

Miller C, Hens M: Multiple sclerosis: a literature review. J Neurosci 1993;25:174–178.

O'Sullivan SB, Schmitz TJ: *Physical Rehabilitation: Assessment and Treatment,* third edition. Philadelphia: Davis, 1994.

Revesz T, Kwon E, Sharer L, Cho E: Multiple sclerosis: pathology of recurrent lesions. Brain 1993;116:681–691.

8

The Case of the Nitroglycerin Episode

You are a home health physical therapist visiting a 72-year-old man who is recovering from an open reduction internal fixation of a right hip fracture. The man has a history of angina and is a non–insulin-dependent diabetic. He is ambulatory with the use of a walker and 50% weight-bearing. He ambulates about his home without difficulty. His improvement in strength and ambulation indicates he has been performing his exercises as requested.

This morning you arrive at his home to find the patient in moderate distress. He indicates that he awoke at about 4:00 a.m. with tightness in the chest and periodic chest pains. He is having slight difficulty with respiration. The patient's pulse while he is supine is about 96 beats per minute. In the same position his blood pressure is 100/70 mmHg. The patient tells you he has taken his medication for diabetes and that his blood sugar levels are within acceptable limits. From the information gathered during the initial evaluation, you are aware that the patient uses nitroglycerin. You ask if he has taken any this morning. He says that he has taken the medication twice since 4:00 a.m. but that it seemed to make no difference in his discomfort. You ask to see the bottle that contains the medication. You note that the nitroglycerin prescription is 2 years old.

What is the appropriate action to take?

RESOLUTION

The therapist contacted emergency medical services, who transferred the patient to the local hospital. In transport the ambulance crew administered additional nitroglycerin. Within moments the patient indicated his chest pain had subsided and that he could breath much easier. After discharge from the hospital it was determined that the nitroglycerin he had been taking was old and ineffective.

DISCUSSION

This patient presented all the symptoms of an acute cardiac event. The therapist attempted to monitor the situation and contacted emergency medical services when conservative measures had failed. The steps taken were appropriate for the situation. The important point in this case is the failure of the nitroglycerin to relieve symptoms. Nitroglycerin relaxes vascular smooth muscle, producing a general vasodilation effect throughout the body. The administration of nitroglycerin has been shown to reduce blood pressure in some patients. Some pharmacists suggest that nitroglycerin pills older than 6 months be discarded.

Therapists who provide home health services need to be aware of the location of medications patients take to help provide the medication in times of distress. Understanding the patient's home environment and how fast acting a prescribed cardiac medication should be assists in determining the severity of a cardiac distress situation.

REFERENCES

Ciccone CD: *Pharmacology in Rehabilitation*. Philadelphia: Davis, 1990.

Eddy L: *Physical Therapy Pharmacology*. St. Louis: Mosby Year Book, 1992.

Loebl S, Spratto GR, Matejski MP, Woods AL: *The Nurse's Drug Handbook*, sixth edition. Delmar, 1991.

Skidmore-Roth L: *Mosby's 1992 Nursing Drug Reference*. St. Louis: Mosby, 1992.

Springhouse Corporation. *Nursing 94 Drug Handbook*. Springhouse, 1994.

9

The Case of the Total Hip Replacement

A 67-year-old man asks that you evaluate his right hip 6 months after total hip replacement surgery. He indicates that he continues to have right leg pain primarily in the anterior mid thigh. According to the patient, he had received extensive post-surgical physical therapy at a rehabilitation center for 1 month. The rehabilitation center provided him with an excellent home program, which he continues to perform with little or no difficulty. With his physician's approval, the patient progressed to working out three times a week at a local fitness center. He walks with no assistive devices.

Upon evaluation, the patient exhibits a limp involving the right lower extremity. The patient reports that pain increases with prolonged ambulation and that his limp seems to worsen the more he ambulates. You find the patient has good range of motion. Strength is not equal to that of the left lower extremity, but there is no evidence of a Trendelenburg deviation that would contribute to the limp. The patient has only minimal soreness on palpation that involves the right hip and thigh. There are no reports of low back pain, and the knee and ankle present full pain-free range of motion. The patient appears frustrated and asks, "I'm returning to my doctor next week. Is there anything I should point out that might be helpful in addressing this problem?"

What are your recommendations?

RESOLUTION

Many patients who have undergone total hip replacement require physical therapy for only a few weeks after the operation. After surgery most patients require assistance primarily with activities of daily living, gait training, and instruction in total hip replacement precautions and exercise. After the operation the goal of the physical therapist is to get the patient moving as quickly as possible by addressing ambulation, bed mobility, and transfers. The therapist also teaches the patient how to maneuver around obstacles in the home. A therapist at a rehabilitation center or a home health physical therapist informs the family about how the patient should progress and teaches them how to enhance progress.

If pain continues in the involved extremity and there is no possibility of a fracture, the therapist examines the patient for possible differences in leg length. In this case the patient presented a difference of approximately ½ inch (12.7 mm), the right leg being shorter than the left. When questioned, the patient replied that he had no idea such a difference in length existed. The therapist who had provided the initial treatment apparently had not informed the patient of the leg length difference. If a true leg length difference is present, the therapist can recommend ordering a shoe lift or shoe insert to correct the problem. Once the device fits properly, additional therapy is seldom required.

DISCUSSION

Despite the efforts of every orthopedic surgeon to ensure leg length equality, obtaining equal leg length can be difficult. Surgeons often inform their patients that every effort will be made to ensure equal length but that steps can be taken after the operation if a difference is present. Many surgeons assess for the presence of a difference in leg length only after several weeks of ambulation. The reason surgeons prefer to wait is that a small difference in leg length may pose no problems to the patient.

REFERENCES

Gogia PP, Christensen CM, Schmidt C: Total hip replacement in patients with osteoarthritis of the hip: improvement in pain and functional status. Orthopaedics 1994;17:145–150.

Goldberg VM: Anatomic cementless total hip replacement: design considerations and early clinical experience. Acta Orthop Belg 1993;59:183–189.

Gorab RS, Covino BM, Borden LS: The rationale for cementless revision total hip replacement with contemporary technology. Orthop Clin North Am 1990;24:627–633.

Guccione AA: *Geriatric Physical Therapy.* St. Louis: Mosby Year Book, 1993.

Hertling D, Kressler RM: *Management of Common Musculoskeletal Disorders: Physical Therapy Principles and Methods,* second edition. Philadelphia: Lippincott, 1990.

10

The Case of the Chronic Smoker

Your patient is a 55-year-old man who was recently hospitalized for a recurring respiratory infection. He was admitted to
the hospital by his family physician after complaining of increased chest congestion, dyspnea, and low-grade fever. The patient has repeatedly reported a persistent mucus-producing
cough that has been present during the winter months for the
past 2 years. He has a long history of heavy cigarette smoking.

The patient reports difficulty with breathing after the slight-
est exertion, even after mild activities of daily living. He can
best be described as being in poor physical condition with a
body weight 20% greater than ideal. His wife describes him as
being very lethargic.

Diagnostic imaging and tests were ordered to assess pulmonary and cardiovascular function. Test results indicated infil-
trates in both lungs, abnormally low pulmonary flow rates
and volumes, an increase in partial pressure of carbon dioxide,
and a decrease in the partial pressure of oxygen in arterial
blood. Electrocardiographic changes in the right side of the
heart were indicative of chronic obstructive pulmonary disease
(COPD).

While hospitalized, the patient received percussion and postural drainage three times a day along with breathing exercises
and incentive spirometry. He received continuous supplemental oxygen at a rate of 2 L/min and was given a low level stress
test. During the test it was determined that the patient could increase his maximum work rate and perform more efficiently if
the oxygen flow were increased to 4 L/min. With antibiotics
and chest physical therapy the respiratory infection resolved,
and the patient was discharged from the hospital. It was the
opinion of the attending physician that the patient would
benefit from continuous supplemental oxygen. An oxygen
concentrator and portable oxygen stroller were ordered for
home use.

Three weeks later the patient was readmitted to the hospital
after several bouts of respiratory arrest. His wife indicated that
whenever he engaged in activities of daily living, which were
stress test–approved, the patient's breathing would become

labored and, at times, cease completely. In addition, the wife indicated the patient would become cyanotic and appear as though he was going to die.

What do you think could be the problem?

RESOLUTION

The patient returned to physical therapy for re-evaluation of exercise tolerance. His exercise capacity was evaluated while he walked with portable oxygen provided by a nasal cannula. Arterial blood gases were monitored indirectly with a pulse oximeter. Results indicated that there had been no clinically significant changes since the last hospitalization. Oxygen and carbon dioxide levels remained stable.

To obtain additional information the therapist questioned the spouse as to the reasons for the sudden episodes of respiratory distress. Information obtained indicated that the patient did well while using the oxygen concentrator but that his condition suddenly deteriorated when the patient used portable oxygen. The therapist next focused on how the oxygen was being administered. The wife said, "When we turn on the oxygen, we always turn it on as high as it will go so he can receive as much as possible." Once the problem was identified (too high a concentration of oxygen) rates were set at 2 L/min at rest and 4 L/min for increased activity levels. The patient was then able to return home without further incident.

DISCUSSION

Patient and family education is an important part of the home therapy regimen of a patient with a chronic pulmonary condition. Patients with COPD have higher levels of carbon dioxide and lower levels of oxygen in their blood than do other people as a result of the pulmonary disease. Patients with COPD gradually adapt physiologically. Unlike the respiratory drive of people with normal lung function, which is triggered by high levels of carbon dioxide, the respiratory drive of patients with COPD depends on low oxygen levels. Increasing the concentration of oxygen actually depresses the respiratory drive of a patient with COPD.

REFERENCES

Frownfelter DL (ed): *Chest Physical Therapy and Pulmonary Rehabilitation: An Interdisciplinary Approach,* second edition. St. Louis: Mosby Year Book, 1987.

Goodman CC, Snyder TEK: *Differential Diagnosis in Physical Therapy: Musculoskeletal and Systemic Conditions.* Philadelphia: Saunders, 1990.

Grant HD, Murray RH, Bergeron JD: *Brady Emergency Care,* fifth edition. Englewood Cliffs: Prentice-Hall, 1990.

Hodgkin JE, Connors CL, Bell CW: *Pulmonary Rehabilitation: Guidelines to Success,* second edition. Philadelphia: Lippincott, 1993.

Ries, AL: Position paper of the American Association of Cardiovascular and Pulmonary Rehabilitation: scientific basis of pulmonary rehabilitation. J Cardiopulmonary Rehabil 1990; 10:418–441.

11

The Case of the Painful Gait

A 45-year-old woman was referred to an outpatient facility after open reduction internal fixation of a left lower extremity tibia-fibula fracture that occurred approximately 4 months ago. The patient had been receiving extensive physical therapy at another facility but her gait had not improved. The fracture is well healed and the patient has been full weight-bearing for approximately 8 weeks. The physical therapist at the other facility has requested a consultation on the case.

Upon evaluation, you note that the patient exhibits an antalgic gait pattern, maintaining the affected foot and ankle in external rotation throughout the gait cycle. The external rotation is most evident during the stance phase of gait. The patient says she is aware her foot turns out and that she limps. The patient says she limps because of pain in the arch that occurs during weight-bearing.

To correct the gait deviation the patient has tried to turn her leg in while walking to position her affected foot like the unaffected side. This reduced the foot pain, but the patient says it feels unnatural and causes pain in the hip and knee after she walks long distances. A muscle test indicates there is minimal strength difference between the two lower extremities and no limitations in range of motion. The patient's symptoms are not reproduced during manual resistive and passive stress tests.

Examination of the foot in full weight-bearing demonstrates the medial longitudinal arch is collapsed in comparison with the uninvolved foot. She wears a foot orthosis, which has provided support to the arch. There is no evidence of a leg length discrepancy.

What could be done to reduce this patient's deviations and pain?

RESOLUTION

The therapist recommended a plastic ankle-foot orthosis with an articulating ankle joint to protect the ankle-foot complex. The ankle-foot orthosis provided definitive three-point pressure control to the rear and midfoot during gait, preventing abnormal compensatory pronation and resultant pain. An articulating ankle joint design was recommended to avoid inhibiting normal ankle dorsiflexion and plantar flexion.

DISCUSSION

It was important to determine the source of abnormal external rotation in the lower extremity. Placing the patient in a short sitting position helped determine that the femoral condyles were parallel to the floor but that the relationship between the ankle malleoli and the femoral condyles exhibited an excessive degree of external torsion.

The patient in this case had suffered a severe compound fracture. During the surgical fixation, the physician was unsuccessful in obtaining proper alignment of the bony structures. The fracture healed in a malaligned position, resulting in an excessive external rotation deformity distal to the fracture site. The pain reported in the foot was attributed to a change in the forces at the foot and ankle joint during the stance phase of gait. The ankle is normally externally rotated approximately 15 degrees in relation to the transverse axis of the knee. Excessive external rotation of the foot and ankle caused the forces, which normally promote dorsiflexion during the stance phase of gait, to contribute to an excessive pronation moment at the foot–ankle complex from heel strike to midstance. This resulted in pain at the medial ankle-foot and an antalgic gait pattern.

In this instance the patient had attempted to compensate by internally rotating the hip. This not only adversely affected the biomechanics of the hip joint but also internally rotated the knee axis relative to the line of progression of walking. Both abnormal compensations were unacceptable, as evidenced by the resultant pain and dysfunction at these joints. The first foot orthosis provided limited benefit because an extrinsic problem (abnormal rotation outside the foot–ankle complex) was the primary cause of the excessive pronation.

REFERENCES

Hunt GC: *Clinics in Physical Therapy,* New York: Churchill Livingstone, 1988.

Norkin CC, Levangie PK: *Joint Structure and Function: A Comprehensive Analysis,* second edition. Philadelphia: Davis, 1992.

Richardson JK, Iglarsh ZA: *Clinical Orthopaedic Physical Therapy.* Philadelphia: Saunders, 1994.

12

The Case of the Weak Knee

An 80-year-old man with arthritis is referred to your facility for postsurgical rehabilitation of a right total knee replacement. The patient arrived in a wheelchair from his home after having been discharged 2 days earlier from a rehabilitation hospital. He required moderate assistance to get out of the car and into a wheelchair. During the transfer the patient indicated he had considerable difficulty maintaining knee extension and that he could not place much weight on the extremity without feeling as though it were going to collapse. The patient first noticed he was having problems with weight-bearing and keeping the knee straight after attempting a pivot transfer into his car after discharge from the rehabilitation hospital.

Upon evaluation, the knee showed swelling not uncommon for a recent total knee replacement. Active-assisted flexion was 100 degrees, and full extension could be attained only while the patient was in the long sitting position. The patient ambulated with a walker and with a very short stride, placing minimal weight on the right lower extremity. He was unable to perform a straight leg raise and demonstrated a very weak quadriceps set that was only palpable in the midquadriceps musculature.

During the next two visits to the clinic, attempts to improve the patient's gait pattern and lessen the presence of a quadriceps lag are unsuccessful. You notice decreased flexibility in the hamstring muscle group and are concerned the patient is not working on his home program.

What would you recommend?

RESOLUTION

It was surmised that, at some point during the transfer into the car at the rehabilitation hospital, the patient sustained a tear of the quadriceps tendon at its insertion. The tear was identified visually and by palpation by requesting the patient to perform a short-arc quadriceps exercise. Although there was virtually no pain while the patient attempted the short arc, very little or no movement could be seen or palpated.

The patient was immediately seen by his orthopedic surgeon. The surgeon advised the patient of the torn tendon and indicated that if a repair were to be made, it would have to be performed within the next several days. If not repaired soon, the tendon would retract to the point where reattachment would be difficult or impossible. Rehabilitation would begin after a long period of immobilization. The knee would have to be in full extension for at least 4 weeks.

In this instance the patient decided not to undergo the repair. The patient said he would prefer to wear a brace rather than endure another operation and rehabilitation. Therapy for the next 2 weeks focused on general conditioning, ambulation, and use of a knee brace to help control knee flexion. The therapist worked toward the goal of independence in ambulation and activities of daily living for the home environment. The patient did quite well throughout the next 2 weeks of daily physical therapy and was discharged as independent with use of a walker.

DISCUSSION

A quadriceps tear is considered rare after total knee replacement. If present, it is usually associated with trauma, such as a fall. When a tear has occurred, repair is best done immediately. After reattachment, the leg must be maintained in full extension for several weeks. Regaining range of motion after these repairs may be difficult. In this case, additional surgical intervention and rehabilitation were avoided by use of a knee orthosis.

REFERENCES

Brashear HR, Raney RB: *Handbook of Orthopedic Surgery*, tenth edition. St. Louis: Mosby, 1986.

Crenshaw AH (ed): *Campbell's Operative Orthopaedics*, eighth edition. St. Louis: Mosby Year Book, 1992.

Rasul JR, Fisher D: Primary repair of quadriceps tendon ruptures. Clin Orthop 1993;289:205–207.

13

The Case of the Normal Radiograph

You receive a call from the podiatry resident asking you to administer a whirlpool to a patient who sought treatment at the podiatry clinic. The patient was initially seen by the podiatry staff 1 week ago because of a painful, draining lesion on the plantar surface of his right foot. He was given oral antibiotics and told to soak the foot in Epsom salts daily. Today, the lesion is still painful and is draining a thin amber-colored fluid. As the patient is brought to you, the podiatry resident explains that a radiograph was obtained and the results were normal. You are asked to give the patient a whirlpool to clean the wound and are asked for a recommendation regarding the care of the patient.

How do you proceed, and what is your recommendation?

RESOLUTION

The patient was cooperative but reported foot pain. The therapist gently placed his foot in the whirlpool and after several minutes began to carefully debride a small amount of necrotic tissue from the lesion. During probing, an object was found deeply embedded in the lesion. Slowly and gently, the therapist removed a thin sliver of wood 2¼ inches long. The therapist placed the sliver in a towel for later inspection and concluded the whirlpool treatment. The patient's foot was removed from the whirlpool, and a wheelchair was used to return the patient to the podiatry clinic. The podiatry staff was surprised to see the sliver of wood. The therapist recommended that the patient use crutches for a few days to limit weight-bearing and facilitate lesion healing.

DISCUSSION

The therapist was correct to treat the wound as described. Use of a whirlpool can be very effective in facilitating tissue debridement. To accurately determine the status of a wound, one must remove necrotic tissue to allow clear visual inspection. Gentle debridement within a whirlpool is often well tolerated by patients and allows considerable cleansing and removal of necrotic tissue and drainage.

It is important to remember that radiographic imaging detects materials such as bone and metal. Wood is not detected with a conventional radiographic examination. When debriding any wound, therapists should carefully search for foreign objects. In this case, the sliver of wood became embedded in the patient's foot while he was walking through a home woodpile wearing only sandals. In addition to the recommendation of using crutches, the therapist could also suggest the patient wear appropriate footwear when going through the woodpile in the future.

REFERENCES

Kloth LC, McCulloch JM, Feeder JA: *Wound Healing: Alternatives in Management*, second edition. Philadelphia: Davis, 1995.

Michlovitz SL: *Thermal Agents in Rehabilitation*, second edition. Philadelphia: Davis, 1990.

Sussman C: Physical therapy modalities and the wound recovery cycle. Ostomy Wound Manage 1992;38:43–51.

14

The Case of the Plant Doctor

For the past several weeks you have been working at a manu-
facturing plant, treating workers and teaching safe work techniques. The plant physician, a retired internist, calls you to
discuss a worker who returned to the job 2 weeks ago. That
worker had been injured 4 months ago when a load of crates
fell from a forklift, pinning his legs. The patient underwent
open reduction internal fixation to repair comminuted fractures
of the tibia and fibula of both lower extremities. His recovery
was rapid and his rehabilitation was accomplished by attending a local exercise club to ride a stationary bike.

The plant physician tells you the worker reports that his left
foot feels tired but not painful after he is on his feet for an hour.
The physician has examined the worker and tells you, "He can
move his feet up and down with his boots on so I know he's
strong. I think he wants more time off work, that's all." The
physician asks you to evaluate the worker and recommend a
course of action.

What do you do?

RESOLUTION

A serious work injury can include a number of complex and sometimes puzzling factors. In this case, the therapist knew the surgical intervention went well and the patient returned to work. The therapist was not sure, however, about the effectiveness of the time spent at the exercise club. He decided to perform a physical therapy evaluation.

The patient's passive range of motion was normal in both lower extremities. Vascular signs also appeared normal. Sensation appeared intact except for the medial aspect of the left foot. The manual muscle test indicated all strengths were normal (5/5) except for the left tibialis anterior muscle. To determine if the patient was truly cooperating, the therapist performed a simple electrodiagnostic test. The test showed that the patient's left tibialis anterior muscle responded only weakly to alternating current, but when stimulated with direct current, the muscle contraction was strong.

The therapist informed the plant physician of the findings, and electromyography (EMG) and nerve conduction velocity (NCV) studies were scheduled. The therapist's suspicions of partial denervation of the tibialis anterior muscle were confirmed. The patient was provided with an ankle orthosis to help reduce the need for muscle substitution by the long toe extensors. Wearing the orthosis, the patient no longer reported foot fatigue and was allowed to return to work. Follow-up EMG and NCV studies were scheduled for the next month.

DISCUSSION

This case outlines the need to carefully evaluate a patient and perform electrodiagnostic tests when problems with sensory or motor nerves are suspected. The worker did not report foot pain and was found to be hyposensitive in the area of the foot associated with the insertion of the involved muscle, the tibialis anterior.

Using alternating as opposed to direct current electrical stimulation is an effective method of determining neurologic injury and reaction to degeneration. Muscle has a longer chronaxie than nerve, which explains why denervated muscle would not respond with a strong contraction to a rapidly alternating current. More prolonged direct current is necessary to stimulate muscle tissue itself.

REFERENCES

Clarkson M, Hazel M, Gulewich GB: *Musculoskeletal Assessment, Joint Range of Motion and Manual Muscle Strength.* Baltimore: Williams & Wilkins, 1989.

Gersh, MR (ed): *Electrotherapy in Rehabilitation.* Philadelphia: Davis, 1992.

Hayes KW: *Manual for Physical Agents,* fourth edition. East Norwalk: Appleton & Lange, 1993.

Kahn J: *Principles and Practice of Electrotherapy,* third edition. New York: Churchill Livingstone, 1994.

Magee DJ: *Orthopedic Physical Assessment,* second edition. Philadelphia: Saunders, 1992.

15

The Case of the Bartender

A 42-year-old bartender has been referred to your clinic by an emergency department physician. The bartender arrived at the emergency department this morning reporting right elbow pain that started 10 days ago, after he worked at a large wedding. The pain prevents the man from uncorking bottles, a task he must frequently perform at work. The emergency department physician ordered radiographs, which were reported as negative for fracture or dislocation of the elbow. The physician then made a diagnosis of inflammation of the radiohumeral joint and prescribed a non-steroidal anti-inflammatory drug. A staff therapist evaluates the patient and notices the elbow is completely painless to palpation and has normal skin temperature and that active range of motion against gravity is normal. Also, resisted elbow flexion is uncomfortable, and resisted supination and flexion are painful and weak. The staff therapist is unsure how to proceed and asks you for assistance.

How do you proceed?

RESOLUTION

The case stimulated a number of questions in the therapist's mind. First, the exact location of the pain was unclear because the elbow is a complex structure that consists of multiple joints and several soft tissues. A diagnosis of joint inflammation in the absence of pain to palpation and an increase in tissue temperature seemed to be inconsistent. Further, why was the diagnosis specific to the radio-humeral joint? Did the pain to resisted flexion and supination implicate that particular joint?

The resolution of this case required clearing the cervical spine and performing a complete upper-quarter screen. Upon evaluation, the therapist noticed the patient's report of pain was not duplicated with palpation. Resisted elbow flexion was uncomfortable, but the combination of resisted elbow flexion and supination caused the patient pain in the elbow and upper arm. Although the radio-humeral joint is involved in that combined motion, the therapist's assessment was that the joint functions were normal. The therapist also noticed that with the elbow extended, the patient described pain in the upper arm as the shoulder was gently hyperextended.

The therapist continued the evaluation, and although it could not be seen, a slight distal shift of the belly of the biceps brachii was palpated as the patient performed resisted elbow flexion and supination. Further analysis demonstrated a partial tear of the tendon of the short head of the biceps. The therapist referred the patient to an orthopedist for possible surgical intervention and informed the emergency department physician of the findings.

DISCUSSION

The patient in this case was injured performing a motion that later became a diagnostic tool. With the origin fixed, the biceps brachii flexes the elbow and supinates the forearm. These were the motions used to uncork bottles. It is important to remember that two joint muscles may require multiple testing positions to rule out involvement. For example, passively extending the elbow and the shoulder helped identify a soft-tissue lesion that was mistaken for a joint problem.

REFERENCES

Crenshaw AH: *Campbell's Operative Orthopedics,* eighth edition. St. Louis: Mosby Year Book, 1992.

Nicholas JA, Hershman BE: *The Upper Extremity in Sports Medicine.* St. Louis: Mosby Year Book, 1990.

Richardson JK, Iglarsh AZ: *Clinical Orthopaedic Physical Therapy.* Philadelphia: Saunders, 1994.

Wilk KE, Andrews JR: *The Athlete's Shoulder.* New York: Churchill Livingstone, 1994.

16

The Case of the Cerebral Vascular Accident

As a home health therapist, you have been treating a 77-year-old woman for 4 weeks. The woman sustained a left cerebral vascular accident (CVA) 6 weeks ago but has experienced a remarkable recovery. She has no motor, sensory, or cognitive deficits. She is independent in all activities of daily living and ambulates on level and elevated surfaces without assistance or an assistive device. The only medication she takes is one aspirin tablet daily.

After a course of therapy conducted in her sister's home, the patient has returned to her own two-story house. You visited the patient in her home during the early evening 2 days ago. She was excited to be back home and demonstrated independence in her surroundings. In fact, she gave you a tour of her home to see the extensive remodeling that had been completed just before her CVA.

One week later you receive a call from the patient's sister. She tells you, "My sister can't use the steps and she seems very confused when I ask where things like her glasses are." The sister explains further, "Events like this occur only in the early afternoon."

The next morning, you stop by the patient's house, finding her weeding the front lawn. You are invited inside and find the patient completely mobile and responding correctly to all questions. She invites you to stay for lunch, and at 1:00 p.m. you decide it is time to leave. You notice, however, that the patient declines to accompany you outdoors and seems unable to tell you why.

Later that afternoon you drive by the patient's house, and she calls and waves to you from the front porch. Again you find her completely mobile and not at all confused. Her sister, who has also stopped by to visit, gently pulls you aside and says, "The doctor was here 15 minutes ago and said she's fine. I guess she's just stubborn and won't do anything right after lunch." However, on the basis of the patient's sister's comments, the physician contacts you and asks for a re-evaluation in the early afternoon to determine the reason for the patient's inconsistent behavior.

How should you approach this re-evaluation?

RESOLUTION

Patient behaviors are based on intricate and complex sets of rules and customs, along with individual experiences, desires, and knowledge. Neurologic disorders such as a CVA can cause changes in many factors, possibly leading to altered patient behavior. At first thought, the therapist might easily have assumed the behaviors described in this case were due to the CVA. The questions the therapist asked are: Why is it only in the early afternoon that the patient's behavior is different? What is specific to that time of day that would cause the patient to be unable to find personal objects (such as glasses) or leave her home?

The therapist conducted a physical therapy evaluation at 1:00 p.m. that did not show any motor or cognitive changes since the last evaluation. The therapist noticed, however, that the patient was unable to locate her glasses on the windowsill, even though she had placed them there only 20 minutes earlier. When the therapist handed the glasses to her, the patient said thank you and donned them correctly. At gait assessment there were no deviations, but the patient adamantly refused to walk down the steps to go outdoors. When asked why not, she simply said, "I'm afraid to."

Because the patient was elderly, the therapist considered the normal changes of aging that may have accounted for the patient's behavior. The therapist also assessed the patient's newly remodeled environment and found it gleaming. The walls and floors were shiny and the home very sunny. It then occurred to the therapist that the bright environment may be associated with the unusual behaviors. For this patient, the solution was a simple one. Curtains were installed to reduce glare from the afternoon sunshine, and the stairwell was modified to eliminate glare from interior lighting.

DISCUSSION

During aging, changes in the eyes render the elderly sensitive to glare. That sensitivity can be exquisite, prohibiting the person from seeing familiar objects or passages. An acute lack of vision can be frightening, causing a patient to avoid behaviors and areas that do not pose problems when glare is not present. With her environment modified to compensate for the normal changes of aging (i.e., elimination of glare to facilitate her vision), the patient in this case resumed normal behavior.

REFERENCES

Bleuclair Group: *Functional Assessment for the Elderly. 1. Cognitive and Special Senses*, New York: New York, 1986.

Cech D, Martin S: *Functional Development Across the Life Span*. Philadelphia: Saunders, 1995.

Christenson MA: Adaptations of the physical environment to compensate for sensory changes. Phys Occup Ther Geriatr 1990;8:3–30.

Hunt L: Aging and the visual system. Insight 1993;18:6–7.

17

The Case of the Troublesome Prosthesis

You are a supervisor of a rehabilitation unit in a hospital setting. One of the staff therapists reports to you in frustration that her patient with a below-knee amputation has a poorly fitting prosthesis that requires immediate attention from the prosthetist. She says that the prosthesis is too long, the suspension is inadequate, and a skin abrasion on the anterior distal tibia has developed. She is angry that such a poorly fitting prosthesis was provided. You calmly assess the situation and ask the therapist if she has performed a comprehensive prosthetic evaluation. She indicates that she has not. Your supervisory recommendation is that you perform the evaluation together before calling the prosthetist.

A review of the patient's history reveals that the patient is a 65-year-old man who underwent a right below-knee amputation 3 weeks ago for a gangrenous ulcer at the ankle secondary to peripheral vascular disease. He has a 15-year history of insulin-dependent diabetes mellitus. The comprehensive patient and prosthetic evaluation demonstrated a number of positive findings. When the patient stood while wearing the prosthesis with equal weight on both lower extremities, the iliac crest on the prosthetic side was approximately 1/2 inch (12.7 mm) higher than the sound side. The prosthetic suspension did appear inadequate as evidenced by excessive pistoning of the prosthesis during the swing phase of gait.

When questioned, the staff therapist reports that she has applied two additional prosthetic socks in an attempt to alleviate the suspension problem. The patient had been experiencing discomfort at the anterior distal tibial area during weight-bearing on the prosthesis. Examination of the residual limb shows a skin abrasion at the anterior distal tibial area. In addition, the weight-bearing mark left by the patellar tendon indentation of the socket is located more distally than expected, presenting over the tibial tubercle rather than the patellar tendon.

What are your recommendations?

RESOLUTION

The initial problem requiring attention in this case was the skin abrasion on the residual limb. The therapists initiated proper wound care procedures and protected the involved area with a thin occlusive dressing during further attempts at use of the prosthesis. The next problem they addressed was the improper position of the residual limb in the prosthetic socket as evidenced by the distal location of the patellar tendon bearing (PTB) weight-bearing mark on the residual limb after the patient used the prosthesis. The therapists removed the prosthetic socks until the residual limb was properly positioned in the socket. They verified the position according to the appropriate location of the PTB weight-bearing mark over the patellar tendon after the patient stood and bore weight on the prosthesis. The therapists did not initiate ambulation until they verified proper residual limb position in the socket and re-checked the skin abrasion for signs of worsening with use of the prosthesis.

The therapists then re-evaluated the height of the prosthesis by comparing the height of the iliac crests while the patient was standing erect with equal weight on both lower extremities and his feet 4 to 6 inches apart. No discrepancy in the height of the iliac crests was noted. The therapists addressed the suspension problem by temporarily placing a wedge of semirigid foam between the prosthetic socket and soft socket insert in the area of the medial suspension wedge. The therapists then consulted the prosthetist about permanent tightening of the medial suspension wedge area.

DISCUSSION

This case illustrates the tendency of some physical therapists to identify and react to the symptoms of prosthetic fitting problems before evaluating and addressing the underlying cause of the problems. The staff therapist addressed the suspension problem by adding prosthetic socks to the residual limb in an attempt to tighten the socket fit. This was an acceptable corrective strategy, but the PTB weight-bearing mark on the residual limb should have been monitored to ensure that the addition of socks did not raise the residual limb out of its proper position in the socket. This mistake contributed to the erroneous conclusion that the prosthesis was too long (the relative leg length discrepancy resulted from the residual limb being positioned too high in the socket) and resulted in an abrasion on the residual limb (the pressure-sensitive areas of the residual limb were no longer matched to the contour and pressure relief areas of the socket). If she had correctly identified that additional prosthetic socks raised the residual limb too high in the socket (the PTB weight-bearing mark would be located below the patella tendon area of the residual limb), the therapist could have concluded that the suspension itself, as opposed to the tightness of the socket, was responsible for the suspension problem.

REFERENCES

Bowker JH, Michael JW: *Atlas of Limb Prosthetics, Surgical Prosthetic, and Rehabilitation Principles*, second edition. St. Louis: Mosby Year Book, 1992.

Karacoloff LA: *Lower Extremity Amputation: A Guide to Functional Outcomes and Physical Therapy Management*. Rockville: Aspen, 1985.

Saunders GT: *Lower Limb Amputations; A Guide to Rehabilitation*. Philadelphia: Davis, 1986.

18

The Case of the 6-year-old Boy

Your patient is a 6-year-old boy with severe mental retardation and low muscle tone, which impairs his gross motor function. He has been ambulating with a rolling walker for about a year and has maintained range within normal limits with active movement available throughout. He has been wearing soft foot orthotics inside both shoes for about a year to help correct a mild pronation problem.

Within the last few months, the patient has stopped using the walker and begun taking some unsupported steps. As the patient's tolerance for this task improves, however, you notice a crouching posture in the lower extremities and an increase in pronation in the feet. Ankle dorsiflexion is available only to neutral with the foot supinated, and pronation is excessive. Other ranges of motion at the hip, knee, and ankle are within normal limits. Active movement remains available at all joints in all planes of movement within available ranges. You refer the child to an orthopedist for an evaluation of these changes in foot and ankle ranges. The orthopedist recommends bilateral tendoachilles lengthening procedures, and the child's mother asks you what you think.

How do you proceed?

RESOLUTION

The therapist considered surgery too drastic for this child, who was just beginning to walk independently—the postoperative immobility would result in loss of skills that had been difficult to gain. The therapist believed a change in orthotics would give the extra correction needed for the pronation problem. She contacted a local orthotist who worked extensively with children, and the orthotist suggested a trial period with supramalleolar orthoses. Both the family and the orthopedist were agreeable to this plan. The therapist was present for the measurement and the delivery of the orthotics and saw almost immediate improvement in hip and knee alignment and a more neutral subtalar position in standing and walking.

Over the next 2 weeks the child was able to wear the orthotics comfortably all day and continued to demonstrate improved lower extremity alignment. He also showed uninterrupted motor development. The therapist included subtalar joint neutral position heelcord stretching in the physical therapy program and taught a home program to the family. The orthopedist was pleased with the child's status after 2 months. He indicated that although heel-cord releases may be needed in the future, he would not recommend surgical intervention at this time.

DISCUSSION

Independent standing and walking place more biomechanical demands on the lower extremities than supported walking. Areas of minor deficit, such as mild pronation, can become amplified when the demands of a task increase. The everted position of the calcaneus allows for shortening of the tendoachilles, which in turn pulls the calcaneus into more eversion. The way to break this cycle is to address the deficits at two joints— limit the pronation at the subtalar joint in weight-bearing and increase the available range of motion at the talocrural joint. Proper orthotic intervention can place the subtalar joint near neutral in standing, and proper alignment of the subtalar joint during heelcord stretching can lead to more selective stretching of the talocrural joint structures. Of course, depending on the amount of deformity, the age and weight of the child, and other factors, different levels of orthotic intervention may be appropriate. One such intervention may include the use of ankle-foot orthoses.

REFERENCES

Donatelli R: *The Biomechanics of the Foot and Ankle.* Philadelphia: Davis, 1990.

Montgomery PC, Connolly BH (eds): *Motor Control and Physical Therapy.* Hixson: Chattanooga Group, 1991.

Orner CE, Turner D, Worrell T: Effect of foot orthoses on the balance skills of a child with a learning disability. Pediatr Phys Ther 1994;6:10–14.

Woollacott MH, Shumary-Cook A: Changes in posture control across the life span: a systems approach. Phys Ther 1990;70:799–807.

19

The Case of the Patient with Paraplegia

Your patient is a 26-year-old woman who has paraplegia at T-9. She describes upper thoracic spinal pain. She has had paraplegia for 5 years from injuries sustained in a motor vehicle accident. The patient is stabilized with Harrington rods to the level of T-5. Symptoms have decreased 50% since treatment began 3 weeks ago. You are able to relieve 90% of the pain with modalities (moist heat, electrical stimulation) and exercise; however, by the next session the pain has again increased to the point that it impedes the patient's ability to maneuver her wheelchair and perform activities of daily living.

Active range of motion is within normal limits for the upper quarter with 4+/5 upper quarter strength. Pain is reproduced on resisted neck extension, shoulder complex elevation, external rotation, horizontal abduction, scapular depression and adduction, and end range rotation of the upper thoracic spine. Pain is most intense in the midspinal region at T3-5. Joint play motion through the cervical and thoracic levels indicates mild hypomobility through the lower cervical levels and hypermobility at T3-4 and T4-5. Pain is reproduced on posterior-anterior glide and rotational-side bend passive motions through T2-5. The patient's functional status is independent, including driving.

You discuss the patient's daily activity, finding nothing that consistently or greatly challenges her cervical or thoracic rotation-side bend or extension. You ask the patient to make a list of her activities from the time she leaves the clinic until she sees you the next evening. You consult with a colleague on the findings but are still puzzled as to the consistent aggravation of the symptoms.

How do you proceed?

RESOLUTION

Apparently the cause of the patient's dysfunction was not being addressed. The therapist made it a point to observe the patient getting into and out of her car, transferring, and entering the building. The therapist noticed the patient had difficulty getting the wheelchair out of the back seat. It occurred to the therapist that the motions the patient performed to remove the wheelchair from the back seat of the car were similar to those that reproduced the symptoms. The therapist's intervention included:

1. Addressing causative factors through patient education and modification of wheelchair removal
2. Treating the mild hypomobility in the lower cervical region, initiating a dynamic stabilization program for the muscles surrounding the upper thoracic spine, and continuing exercise to strengthen and increase the endurance of the thoracic and scapular muscles
3. Continuing the use of modalities as appropriate to the stage of healing

DISCUSSION

One of the reasons this patient's symptoms continued was that the causative factors had not been addressed. The modalities and exercise appeared to have a positive effect on the soft tissues and likely relieved some of the inflammation of secondary structures involved. However, the hypermobility at T3-4 and T4-5 remained, and the soft tissue continued to be irritated when this region was challenged. The activity of getting the wheelchair out of the car excessively stressed this region. This injury likely occurred over time with the combined factors of repetitive motion, biomechanical changes, and high stress. Therapists must remember that for patients whose spines are stabilized, the biomechanics of removing a wheelchair from a car can increase stress on vertebral levels proximal to the stabilization.

REFERENCES

Goodman CC, Snyder TEK: *Differential Diagnosis in Physical Therapy*. Philadelphia: Saunders, 1990.

Kendall FP, McCreary EK: *Muscles, Testing and Function*. Baltimore: Williams & Wilkins, 1993.

Saunders HD, Saunders R: *Evaluation, Treatment and Prevention of Musculoskeletal Disorders*, third edition. Vol 1, *Spine*. Bloomington: Saunders & Saunders, 1993.

20

The Case of Low Back Pain

You evaluate a 45-year-old man who reports right-sided low back pain of nontraumatic onset about 2 weeks ago. He has a 5-year history of intermittent low back pain resulting initially from a lifting injury. He is employed as a driver for a postal delivery service. The patient describes his pain as constant, varying in intensity from 3 to 6 out of 10 (0 = no pain, 10 = worst pain). The patient has tried his usual remedy of rest, moist heat, and stretching, but this has not reduced his symptoms, and the pain has increased over the past few days.

The patient's sitting posture during the interview changes constantly, and discomfort is evident. Standing posture reveals slight right-side bend and reduced lumbar concavity. Forward bend and backward bend are mildly restricted but do not alter the symptoms. Left-side bend and rotation are limited and cause a pulling-stretching sensation through the right trunk but do not alter the original symptoms. Lower extremity and neurologic screens are unremarkable. A spring test over the lower thoracic and upper lumbar vertebrae increases the patient's pain, and palpation of the posterolateral trunk region just inferior to the right rib cage elicits increased discomfort and considerable tenderness.

What are your concerns?

RESOLUTION

The therapist's primary concern was an inability to reproduce the pain through mechanical evaluation of the lumbosacral region except for the spring test and palpation of the right posterolateral trunk region. Answers to additional questions about the onset of symptoms and medical history revealed that the back pain is generally brought on by lifting at work. However, this bout with pain was unrelated to any specific activity. The pain this time was constant, and the patient was unable to relieve the pain by altering his position. He also reported that the pain was worse at night and when he was voiding. He denied any recent illness but reported that he had felt fatigued over the past few weeks.

The therapist did not initiate treatment in light of the findings. She discussed the findings with the patient and strongly recommend that he seek medical attention as soon as possible. The therapist offered to make the initial contact with the patient's physician and to follow up with a written report of the findings.

This patient's condition was subsequently diagnosed as pyelonephritis. He returned to the clinic to undergo treatment of his recurring lumbosacral dysfunction in the form of education, body mechanics training, and a home conditioning and exercise program.

DISCUSSION

This case demonstrates the need for a thorough evaluation that includes taking a complete history and asking questions pertaining to systemic illness. In light of the changing health care environment and the fact that many physical therapists now practice without referral and have the legal ability to evaluate without referral, the need for comprehensive evaluation has been brought to the forefront in the professional literature. Therapists who serve as primary health care providers must be able to screen for underlying disease and make decisions regarding referral and appropriate function within their scope of practice. In this case physical therapy may have ill-served the patient.

REFERENCES

Goodman CC, Snyder TEK: *Differential Diagnosis in Physical Therapy.* Philadelphia: Saunders, 1990.

Porterfield JA, DeRosa C: *Mechanical Low Back Pain: Perspectives in Functional Anatomy.* Philadelphia: Saunders, 1990.

Saunders HD, Saunders R: *Evaluation, Treatment and Prevention of Musculoskeletal Disorders*, third edition. Vol 1, *Spine.* Bloomington: Saunders & Saunders, 1993.

21

The Case of Degenerative Disk Disease

A colleague consults you about a 56-year-old woman who reports right-sided cervical and right shoulder and arm pain. After 2 weeks of treatment there has been minimal improvement. The referral from an orthopedic surgeon provides a diagnosis of degenerative disk disease of the cervical spine. The history is insidious onset starting 6 months ago. Radiographs indicate severe degenerative disk disease of the lower cervical spine with narrowing, lipping, and osteophytes at C4-7. Your colleague has performed an evaluation and found limitation in all cervical motions with reproduction of the cervical pain during active right rotation, right lateral bend, and extension. The postural analysis revealed severe forward head posture, exaggerated thoracic kyphosis, and rounded shoulders. The patient reports tenderness to palpation in the right cervical region as well as in the right upper trapezius and posterior right shoulder. Initial treatment included moist heat, ultrasound, manual cervical traction, active range of motion, and soft-tissue massage to the cervical region.

As part of your evaluation you note that active range of motion is restricted by pain only during rotation to the right with all other restrictions secondary to joint or soft-tissue limitations. Passive range of motion of the cervical spine is restricted by joint or soft-tissue limitations, especially in the lower cervical levels. It does not, however, reproduce pain. Compression–distraction tests of the cervical spine have been unremarkable.

You look at the shoulder complex and find that active range of motion is within normal limits. However, mid- to end range active external rotation, elevation, and extension reproduce the symptoms. You notice that the patient's movement pattern for elevation of the shoulder is asymmetric, the right upper shoulder complex demonstrating abnormal scapular elevation. Strength testing reveals weakness of external rotators and extensors because of pain. Palpation reveals hyperactivity and tenderness of the right cervical muscles and upper trapezius and tenderness at the posterior aspect of the glenohumeral joint extending through the infraspinatus fossa.

On further questioning you learn that the symptoms are aggravated by work. The patient has been employed as a secretary at a local school district for 24 years. Seven months ago her responsibilities changed to include contacting substitute teachers and performing all photocopying for a middle school. The patient indicates she cradles the phone against her right shoulder while utilizing right cervical lateral bend and isometric scapular elevation. She is right-handed and performs repetitive shoulder horizontal abduction and external rotation motions at the copier for what amounts to 2 or more hours a day.

What are your recommendations to your colleague?

RESOLUTION

The therapist suggested that the colleague address the causative factors through patient education and modification of work activities. That posture and work activities contributed to the dysfunction made modification of such activities vital to the plan of care. The therapist also suggested that the colleague direct treatment toward all involved tissues with modalities, therapeutic exercise, and manual soft-tissue techniques appropriate to the stage of healing. The therapist also suggested that the colleague tell the patient to avoid pain-producing activities.

DISCUSSION

Additional and more comprehensive evaluation revealed that a strain of the right cervical muscles and the external rotators and extensors of the shoulder was the primary cause of discomfort. If the patient's symptoms were solely related to degenerative disk disease of the cervical spine (assuming accompanying radicular pain), one would expect that stressing the cervical tissues would have reproduced the shoulder pain as well. Looking for other causative factors or dysfunctions reinforces the importance of individual evaluation and physical therapy diagnosis.

Additional questioning about the patient's symptoms and activities lent additional information to the case. Careful questioning of the patient can reveal the cause of dysfunction. If the patient continued to repeatedly traumatize the involved soft tissue through postural stress and work activities, the best physical therapy would have only limited results. Symptom remediation cannot be achieved without consideration of daily biomechanical stresses and the patient's ability to handle them. Using modalities such as pulsed ultrasound to treat the inflammation and speed the patient into the proliferative phase of healing is appropriate. Therapeutic exercise may include pain-free isometrics and active range of motion. Manual soft-tissue treatment may include massage or myofascial techniques.

REFERENCES

Cyriax JH, Cyriax PJ: *Illustrated Manual of Orthopaedic Medicine.* Boston: Butterworth-Heinemann, 1983.

Magee DJ: *Orthopaedic Physical Assessment,* second edition. Philadelphia: Saunders, 1992.

Richardson JK, Iglarsh ZA: *Clinical Orthopaedic Physical Therapy.* Philadelphia: Saunders, 1994.

22

The Case of Poor Posture

You are a staff physical therapist at a rehabilitation hospital. A colleague consults you about a patient, seen in the outpatient facility, who has a diagnosis of amyotrophic lateral sclerosis (ALS). This 40-year-old man was referred for aquatic physical therapy to improve his ambulatory ability after a right tibial fracture sustained as the patient was entering a limited-access doorway at work. The patient's pain and fatigue have responded to therapeutic exercise in a warm, buoyant environment. Despite the improvement, however, functional progress is limited by shortness of breath.

Review of this case shows that this previously healthy, ambulatory man has experienced progressive neurodegenerative changes over a 3-year period. The patient's neurologist has expressed concern regarding the imposition of disuse atrophy on an already weakened musculoskeletal system. Physical examination is remarkable for clear breath sounds, diminished vital capacity and tidal volume, intact gag reflex without history of aspiration, intact speech with slightly diminished volume, a weak, nonproductive cough, and a resting respiratory rate of 22 to 24 breaths per minute. The patient sacral sits in his motorized scooter with forward head, rounded shoulders with winged scapulae, increased cervical-thoracic kyphosis, and unsupported upper extremities. Standing with a walker reveals pronounced proximal muscle weakness requiring the patient to lock-out his shoulders and elbows while stabilizing an anteriorly tilted pelvis with maximally stretched Y ligaments and hyperextended knees. The patient's abdomen is protuberant, and he reports frequent bouts of low back pain.

How do you help this patient?

RESOLUTION

In the absence of primary pulmonary disease the therapist addressed the musculoskeletal contributions to the patient's increased work of breathing. Recommendations included diaphragmatic, segmental, and pursed-lip breathing exercises and incentive spirometry; gentle stretching of tight pectoral muscles; adaptation of the motorized scooter with an appropriate seat cushion, lumbar roll, and elevated arm rests; use of a combined lumbar corset–abdominal binder; and energy conservation and activity-pacing techniques with use of the Borg scale and dyspnea index. With the exception of the equipment modifications, all these recommendations were adapted for use with the aquatic physical therapy regimen.

DISCUSSION

ALS is a progressive neurodegenerative disease that causes varying patterns of muscle weakness and atrophy combined with spasticity and hyper-reflexia. Death usually occurs within 3 to 6 years of onset, most commonly because of respiratory insufficiency or infection. The patient in this case was a man who, because of relatively slow disease progression and intensive rehabilitative efforts, had remained functionally independent and working until the time of his lower extremity fracture. The resulting immobility and disuse atrophy diminished the patient's independence and his ability to work. Of greater threat, however, were the potential sequelae of immobility and decreased functional residual capacity. These problems lead to early airway closure and ventilation-perfusion mismatching, increased blood viscosity, and venous pooling.

Aquatic exercise addressed the musculoskeletal problems as they related to functional mobility, transfers, standing balance, and ambulation. The patient remained limited in his functional abilities because of a number of unsolved problems that contributed to his increased work of breathing. These problems included ventilatory muscle weakness (diaphragm, abdominal muscles, cervical-thoracic paraspinal muscles, serratus anterior muscle) and tightness (pectoral muscles), slumped posture with compromised thoracic expansion, and inability to pace activities for fatigue and dyspnea management. An elevated resting respiratory rate provided a natural compensation to improve oxygen delivery while simultaneously reinforcing the patient's perception of increased respiratory effort.

Breathing exercises, combined with cervical-thoracic stretching techniques, addressed the ventilatory muscle and thoracic expansion deficits. In this patient's case, some gains in muscle strength were documented, presumably as a reversal of his recent acute immobility. Because of the progressive nature of ALS, passive techniques such as seating modifications and the use of an abdominal binder serve as external contributors to breathing efficiency. A seating system that facilitates a neutral, upright posture with easily fixed upper extremities allows for improved thoracic expansion with assistance from accessory ventilatory muscles. The binder provides increased compression of the abdominal contents with cephalad displacement of the diaphragm. This modification improved the length-tension relationship of the dome-shaped muscle. Inspiratory capacity, vital capacity, and tidal volume were subsequently enhanced.

Use of energy conservation and pacing techniques with visual guides such as the Borg and dyspnea scales provided the patient with structured activity guidelines adaptable to any functional level or activity. These changes in his aquatic therapy regimen facilitated the patient's return to household-level ambulation.

REFERENCES

American College of Sports Medicine: *Guidelines for Exercise Testing and Prescription,* fourth edition. Malvern: Lea & Febiger, 1991.

Cantu RC (ed): *Neurology in Primary Care.* New York: MacMillan, 1985.

Frownfelter DL: *Chest Physical Therapy and Pulmonary Rehabilitation,* second edition. Chicago: Year Book, 1987.

Weiner WJ (ed): *Neurology for the Non-Neurologist,* second edition. Philadelphia: Lippincott, 1989.

Zadai CC: *Pulmonary Management in Physical Therapy.* New York: Churchill Livingstone, 1992.

23

The Case of a New Diagnosis

You are asked to evaluate an 87-year-old man who has returned to the nursing home from the hospital with a diagnosis of acute cerebral vascular accident (CVA). He was admitted to the nursing home 2 years ago because of short-term memory problems. He had been alert, oriented to person, place, and time, and independent in mobility and all activities of daily living, including management of eyeglasses, hearing aids, and dentures. The patient began experiencing problems with these activities about 1 week ago and was hospitalized. The referring physician has requested that a physical therapist evaluate and treat the patient.

Upon evaluation, you find the patient to be alert, but he gives inappropriate answers to most questions. He is able to follow commands with use of visual cuing. Range of motion and strength are within normal limits throughout and equal bilaterally. Bed mobility is independent. The patient can maintain a seated position unassisted. When standing, the patient requires minimal assistance of one to prevent losing his balance. He also requires minimal assistance with bed-to-chair transfers because of balance problems and lack of safety awareness. Gait is unsteady and ataxic. Moderate assistance is required for safe ambulation.

What more should be assessed before you initiate treatment?

RESOLUTION

The physical therapist found the lack of conclusive evidence of a CVA confounding. That the patient could accurately follow visual but not verbal cues was an inconsistency. The patient's hearing aids were checked and found to be full of wax. It was then discovered that the patient's ears were blocked with wax. When the hearing aids and the patient's ears were cleaned, there was an immediate 100% recovery.

DISCUSSION

There was no evidence that this patient suffered a CVA. These findings were supported by a normal electroencephalogram, computed tomographic scan, and magnetic resonance image. The diagnosis had apparently been made purely on the basis of clinical signs and symptoms. The patient presented with confusion, balance abnormalities, and a gait disturbance—all clinical manifestations of a CVA. Alternatives to a CVA had apparently been overlooked.

It is important to recognize that there may be problems with hearing aids or glasses, there may be an electrolyte imbalance that causes symptoms similar to a CVA, or medication may affect a person adversely, causing symptoms similar to those found in people with true CVAs. Sensory changes also may precipitate balance dysfunction corresponding to a CVA. To prevent problems such as these, ears and hearing aids should be examined for cleanliness and function every month.

REFERENCES

Blair FE: *Alzheimers, Stroke, and 29 Other Neurological Disorders Sourcebook*. Detroit: Omnigraphics, 1993.

Lang NM, Kraegel JM, Rantz MJ, Krejci JW: *Quality of Healthcare for Older People in America: A Review of Nursing Studies*. Milwaukee: University of Wisconsin School of Nursing, 1990.

O'Sullivan SB, Schmitz TJ: *Physical Rehabilitation: Assessment and Treatment*, third edition. Philadelphia: Davis, 1994.

24

The Case of the Bilateral Hip Replacements

A 75-year-old woman is referred by her family physician for physical therapy for heat and strengthening exercises to relieve left hip pain. The patient had bilateral total hip replacements for severe degenerative joint disease—the left 1 year ago, the right 2 years ago. Her history also includes a quadruple coronary artery bypass 6 years ago. During evaluation, the patient reports that she has frequent bouts of left hip pain and left leg weakness. She denies cardiac symptoms. Pain in the left hip is 6 out of 10 (0 = no pain, 10 = worst pain) and has been constant for approximately 2 weeks.

Upon evaluation, you find that both hips exhibit mild adhesive scarring anteriorly and laterally. Using a modified Thomas test you determine the patient has bilateral hip flexion contractures of approximately 5 degrees. Hip strength is grossly 4/5 bilaterally. Knee and ankle strength are within functional limits except for left ankle dorsiflexion, which is 3/5. Sensation appears to be intact in both lower extremities.

What else needs to be assessed before you treat this patient?

RESOLUTION

The therapist assessed joints proximal to the hip. Upon evaluation of the lumbosacral spine, severe limitation of range of motion and increased pain were exhibited during forward flexion, extension, left-side bending, and left rotation. Limitation of range of motion was also evident during right-side bending and right rotation. The L-4 reflex was diminished. Straight leg raise was limited more on the left than the right. To ascertain the presence of any additional problems, the therapist referred the patient for diagnostic imaging of the spine before initiation of physical therapy. Imaging revealed a tumor at L3-4 compressing the spinal cord.

DISCUSSION

Frequently, leg pain is the symptom of back problems and can be effectively treated with physical therapy. However, in the case of this patient, if it had been assumed that the pain was caused by tight hip flexors or other soft-tissue restriction (which is a likely scenario) harm could have been done with incorrect treatment. The history of 2 weeks of steady pain, weak left ankle dorsiflexion, and left hip pain combined to warn the alert therapist that there may be other problems.

REFERENCES

Borgquist L, Nilsson LT, Lindelow G, Wilklund I, Thorngren KG: Health policy and musculoskeletal condition. Curr Opin Rheumatol 1992;4:167–173.

Brismar B, Veress B, Svensson O: Injury of the femoral artery in total hip replacements causing abdominal pain and hypovolemic shock. J Bone Joint Surg [Am] 1992;74:1560–1562.

Cyriax JH, Cyriax PJ: *Illustrated Manual of Orthopaedic Medicine*. Boston: Butterworth-Heinemann, 1983.

Fumero S, Dettoni A, Gallinaro M, Crova M: Thigh pain in cementless hip replacement. Ital J Orthop Traumatol 1992;18:167–172.

Goodman CC, Snyder TEK: *Differential Diagnosis in Physical Therapy*. Philadelphia: Saunders, 1990.

Magee DJ: *Orthopedic Physical Assessment*, second edition. Philadelphia: Saunders, 1992.

Olehsak M, Edge AJ: Compression of the sciatic nerve by methylmethacrylate cement after total hip replacement. J Bone Joint Surg 1992;74:729–730.

Richardson JK, Iglarsh ZA: *Clinical Orthopedic Physical Therapy*. Philadelphia: Saunders, 1994.

Salman M, Taylor DC, Beauchamp CP, Duncan CP: Prevention of vascular injuries in revision total hip replacement. Can J Surg 1992;35:261–264.

25

The Case of the Bathroom Spill

You have been treating a 55-year-old woman with right upper extremity paralysis and right lower extremity paresis as an outpatient for 2 months. She sustained a middle cerebral artery hemorrhage 4 months ago. Lower extremity strength, function, and control have improved from flaccid to the poor-fair range. Sensation in the lower extremity is dulled. Upper extremity strength remains zero with minimal flexor tone. Sensation is essentially absent in the right upper extremity. The family has been instructed in upper and lower extremity range of motion and guarding for safe transfers with excellent carry-over.

The patient has never reported any pain previously. Today she describes rib pain. Your evaluation reveals intense right posterolateral thoracic pain with passive right shoulder movement. There is tenderness in the right axilla, and palpation of the right supraspinatus muscle reproduces the pain. Pain also increases with sneezing or coughing. Upon questioning, you learn that the patient had fallen in the bathroom onto her right side 2 days ago. Radiographs of the ribs had been taken and were normal.

What do you do?

RESOLUTION

The therapist immediately stopped ranging the right shoulder and requested a radiograph of the right upper quadrant. Pain was exacerbated by shoulder movement and sudden chest movement. There was also pain on palpation of the supraspinatus muscle and tenderness in the right axilla. The new radiograph revealed a fracture involving the right scapula.

DISCUSSION

After a cerebral vascular accident, especially when sensation is impaired, pain often can be referred. In this case, the patient felt pain in the region adjacent to the actual fracture. However, there are times when pain can be referred away from the injury site and is worthy of assessment because it can indicate a serious problem.

Because the pain was felt in the posterolateral thoracic area, the initial radiographs did not include the scapula at an angle at which the fracture could be identified. Attention was being directed at the ribs, where the pain was perceived; the scapula may have been overlooked in the original radiograph.

When there is a fall in a confined area, it is often difficult to assess what, if anything, the person struck during the accident. The patient's final resting position after the fall should be carefully noted as should any objects in the path of descent. Pain on coughing and sneezing may be a manifestation of several disorders, such as herniation of a disc or fracture of a rib, scapula, or the sternum.

REFERENCES

Bohannon RW, Andrews AW: Shoulder subluxation and pain in stroke patients. Am J Occup Ther 1990;44:507–509.

Culham E, Peat M: Functional anatomy of the shoulder complex. J Orthop Sports Phys Ther 1993;18:342–350.

Joynt RL: The source of shoulder pain in hemiplegia. Arch Phys Med Rehabil 1992;73:409–413.

Martin SD, Weiland AJ: Missed scapular fracture after trauma: a case report and a 23 year follow-up report. Clin Orthop 1994;299:259–260.

Neeman RL, Liederhouse JJ, Neeman M: A multidisciplinary efficacy study on orthokinesis treatment of a patient with post-CVA hemiparesis and pain. Can J Rehabil 1988;2:41–53.

Richardson JK, Iglarsh ZA: *Clinical Orthopedic Physical Therapy.* Philadelphia: Saunders, 1994.

Totta M, Beck G: Shoulder dysfunction in stroke hemiplegia. Phys Med Rehabil Clin North Am 1991;2:627–641.

Wood C: Shoulder pain in stroke patients. Nurs Times 1989;85:32–34.

26

The Case of a Need to Ambulate

A previously independent 68-year-old woman was admitted to your acute care facility 1 week ago with a peptic ulcer and gastrointestinal bleeding. Her only remarkable medical history includes peripheral vascular disease. The physician requests your intervention to evaluate and mobilize this woman in preparation for discharge in the morning.

Your assessment indicates the patient has 3-3.5/5 muscle strength in all extremities. She is independent in bed mobility. The patient states she has, in the past, experienced edema of her feet and ankles due to the peripheral vascular disease. This has not, however, interfered with her mobility. She has been able to ambulate 1/2 mile without lower extremity discomfort. The patient does not express discomfort while sitting and has a blood pressure reading of 120/80 mmHg. As soon as she stands, however, she experiences a syncopal episode with a drop in blood pressure to 90/56 mmHg and a heart rate decrease from 75 to 50 beats per minute. After the patient sits for 3 to 5 minutes and has a blood pressure return to 120/80 mmHg, you attempt to stand the patient a second time. The patient again experiences a syncopal episode with a drop in blood pressure to 86/58 mmHg and a heart rate decrease to 54 beats per minute.

What are your recommendations?

RESOLUTION

Mobilization is important for patients who have been on bed rest and are preparing to return home. In this case, the patient had poor venous return caused by a combination of bed rest and peripheral vascular disease. After the therapist fitted the patient with compression stockings, the patient did not have any clinically significant changes in vital signs or syncope when she stood. The therapist deduced that application of compression stockings helped prevent accumulation of blood and fluid in the lower extremities, alleviating syncopal episodes and allowing mobilization. In this case, the stockings allowed the patient to participate in a program of progressive mobilization, and she returned home. After several days of home health physical therapy, the patient was able to discontinue use of the stockings.

DISCUSSION

Syncope is a transient form of unconsciousness. Causes of syncope may be a drop in blood pressure due to vasodilatation of peripheral vessels and reduced venous return. In postural syncope, failure of normal vasoconstrictive mechanisms contribute to inadequate blood flow to the brain. Compression stockings help prevent venous accumulation in the lower extremities and assist venous return.

REFERENCES

Campbell AD: Pneumatic compression stockings: preventing deep vein thrombus and pulmonary embolus. Today OR Nurse 1990;12:28–29.

Herzog, JA: Deep vein thrombosis in the rehabilitation client: diagnostic tools, prevention, and treatment modalities. Rehabil Nurs 1993;18:67–68.

O'Sullivan SB, Schmitz TJ: *Physical Rehabilitation: Assessment and Treatment*, third edition. Philadelphia: Davis, 1994.

Smith K: Preventing postoperative venous thrombosis: graduated compression stockings. Nurs Mirror 1985;160:29–30.

27

The Case of the Runner

You are consulted to evaluate a 19-year-old female college freshman who is a long-distance runner. She began to develop posteromedial and distal tibial pain approximately 7 weeks ago, which initially occurred only during running and was diagnosed as posteromedial shin splints. She had increased her mileage from 20 miles per week to 35 miles per week when she arrived at college, which was 9 weeks ago. Her pain has continued to increase over the past 3 weeks, and she has been treated by the university athletic training department with rest, ice, compression, and elevation (RICE) for the past 4 weeks. She has noted minimal improvement.

During your evaluation you find her pain present even during walking and that the patient has been unable to practice with the team for the past 3 weeks. The patient's leg is tender to palpation over the distal posteromedial tibia. No neurologic signs or deficits are present, though the patient does report tightness and pressure in her lower leg when she runs. Radiographs and a bone scan have been obtained, both of which were normal. You are asked to initiate treatment based on the above findings.

What are your recommendations?

RESOLUTION

This case demonstrates a need for careful differentiation between conditions that present similarly but respond to different treatments. The therapist determined that the problem was posterior compartment syndrome (increased tissue fluid pressure in a closed fascial space, compromising circulation to nerves and muscles) rather than posteromedial shin splints. These two conditions have many similarities; however, careful evaluation of the signs and symptoms can help one differentiate between them.

The therapist changed the patient's treatment to include frequent (4 times a day) stretching of the muscles of the lower extremity, especially the posterior tibial muscles; soft-tissue mobilization (3 to 4 times a week); and proper warm-ups before running. The therapist prescribed a warm-up that consisted of 20 minutes of stretching, gentle soft-tissue mobilization of the affected area, 10 to 15 minutes of stationary bike riding at a slow pace, and 2 miles of running at a slow (9 minutes per mile) pace. The problem began to resolve, and 4 weeks after the initiation of treatment, the patient was running 30 miles a week pain free. Long warm-up periods and performing activities at a level that did not cause any symptoms were the key to recovery. After 6 weeks using her new regimen, the patient had returned to running 35 miles a week and performing all required team workouts, including track work and running hills.

DISCUSSION

Shin splints tend to respond to RICE, and the pain is more commonly described as a stabbing or sharp pain. Posterior compartment syndrome commonly involves pressure or a cramping in the affected area. Possible clinical presentations may include tingling and occasional muscle weakness, such as foot drop (seen in anterior compartment syndrome). Elevated pressure in the involved compartment, compared with the uninvolved extremity, is commonly found. This increase in pressure results in compression of neural and vascular structures.

REFERENCES

D'Ambrosia RD, Drez D: *Prevention and Treatment of Running Injuries*, second edition. Thorofare: Slack, 1989.

Hutchinson MR, Ireland ML: Common compartment syndromes in athletes: treatment and rehabilitation. Sports Med 1994;17:200–208.

Manoli A, Fakhouri AJ, Weber TG: Concurrent compartment syndromes of the foot and leg. Foot Ankle 1993;14:339–342.

28

The Case of the Headache

You receive a referral to evaluate a 34-year-old woman who has been experiencing headaches for 2 years. She reports some fluctuation in the pain level, but never more than 1 to 2 days of total remission from pain. She also reports right shoulder and neck pain associated with the headaches. Her pain would commonly become worse during the day at her job, a secretarial position, which she has not been able to perform for the past 4 months because of pain. She reports only a minimal reduction in pain since leaving work. The headaches sometimes awaken the patient at night, and the patient is aware she grinds her teeth while sleeping.

The patient has seen her family physician, a specialist in headache disorders and migraines, a psychologist, and a chiropractor with no relief of symptoms. She has also developed irritable bowel syndrome in the past year. Because of the intestinal disorder, the patient has been reluctant to take medication to control her headaches because she believes the headache medication contributes to the abdominal pain. The patient can relate no trauma or incident to the origin of the headaches.

Magnetic resonance images and radiographs have revealed no abnormalities. During your evaluation you find grossly limited cervical range of motion, faulty posture and associated muscle imbalances, and pain over the temporomandibular joints (TMJ) with jaw motion and palpation. You are able to reproduce the shoulder pain and intensify the headache with provocative testing of the cervical spine.

What are your recommendations?

RESOLUTION

This patient presented with cervical spine and TMJ dysfunction. Treatment consisted of cervical spine mobilization (most involved at O-A but hypomobile from C1-5), manual traction to elongate the cervical and associated tissues, and exercises to improve upper quarter range of motion and postural alignment. Education regarding posture during activities of daily living, and moist heat to treat components of the dysfunction such as muscle spasm also were included.

The TMJ dysfunction (anterior disk dislocation with reduction) was addressed through exercise, modalities (ultrasound and electrical stimulation) to decrease her pain, and education. The patient was seen by a dentist specializing in TMJ dysfunction, who fitted her for an oral appliance. The patient returned to work within 2 months. When discharged from physical therapy at the end of 3 months, the patient reported an 80% decrease in abdominal symptoms related to irritable bowel syndrome. She attributed the improvement to decreased stress now that she was recovering.

DISCUSSION

With a program of exercise, joint mobilization, modalities to decrease pain, and patient education, the patient was able to quickly achieve a decrease in pain and a return to a functional lifestyle. This case demonstrates that many health care providers do not fully understand that cervical spine or TMJ dysfunction should be suspected in cases of head and face pain. Even after this patient reported cervical and shoulder pain and nocturnal bruxism, TMJ dysfunction was overlooked. In the physical therapy evaluation, headaches and occipital pain made worse by provocative testing of the cervical spine and that respond quickly to treatment of cervical spinal dysfunction (grade II mobilization to decrease pain) should lead one to believe that headaches may originate from the cervical spine. Provocative testing of the structures that could be involved is important to determine the cause of the pain and whether or not physical therapy is appropriate.

REFERENCES

Calliet R: *Head and Face Pain Syndromes.* Philadelphia: Davis, 1992.

Magee DJ: *Orthopedic Physical Assessment,* second edition. Philadelphia: Saunders, 1992.

Richardson JK, Iglarsh ZA: *Clinical Orthopaedic Physical Therapy.* Philadelphia: Saunders, 1994.

29

The Case of the Iliotibial Band Syndrome

You receive a referral to evaluate a 25-year-old woman triathlete who reports right lateral knee pain of 3 months duration. She has been referred with a diagnosis of iliotibial band (ITB) friction syndrome. The patient's physician treated her with oral anti-inflammatory medication and gave her a cortisone injection into the tissue below the ITB. Neither of these interventions reduced the pain.

The patient has been unable to ride a bicycle or run for the past 2 months because of the pain. She swims 6 days a week, which does not cause pain, and exercises on a cross-country ski simulator every day. By not flexing her knee more than 25 degrees on the ski simulator, the patient avoids pain.

Upon evaluation, you find point tenderness of the ITB over the lateral epicondyle of the femur, which is greatest at approximately 30 degrees of knee flexion. You observe that the patient's right knee is in excessive varus and that the right foot pronates during gait. The patient relates that before the pain began, she had been increasing mileage in both bicycling and running in preparation for a triathlon.

What are your recommendations?

RESOLUTION

The therapist identified the factors causing the ITB friction syndrome, such as inflexibility, and the patient gradually returned to activity at a pain-free level. The therapist provided the patient with a stretching program emphasizing the ITB, hamstrings, and gastrocnemius muscles. Ultrasound to the ITB was used to increase extensibility, followed by soft-tissue mobilization of the tensor fascia lata and ITB. Increasing the length of the ITB with a stretching program is an integral part of reducing the friction that occurs as the ITB passes over the lateral epicondyle of the femur.

The patient began a gradual return to running and biking, at a level that did not reproduce symptoms, 3 weeks into her treatment. The patient performed ice massage on herself after running and biking. An orthotic (a medial wedge) was fabricated to control the excess pronation. Excessive pronation at the subtalar joint can cause internal rotation of the tibia, which increases tension on the ITB.

DISCUSSION

Competitive athletes often try to resume their previous level of activity and intensity as soon as their pain decreases. As a result, they typically suffer recurrences of pain and inflammation, leading to a chronic inflammatory process. Though athletes commonly stretch, the amount of stretching is usually not sufficient to change the tissue length appreciably. This patient was treated successfully with a combination of modalities, stretching, and orthotics.

ITB friction syndrome can frequently be traced to training errors. Weakness in hip musculature may contribute to ITB friction syndrome as the forces absorbed by the ITB increase. Another point to consider is that running shoes should not be worn past their normal wear cycle (400 to 500 miles). Runners should be careful on cambered roads, switching sides of the road so as not to produce an artificial genu varum. There are many possible causes of ITB friction syndrome, and identifying and correcting them is critical to prevent recurrence.

REFERENCES

Aronen G, Chronister R, Regan K, Henisen MA: Practical, conservative management of iliotibial band syndrome. Phys Sports Med 1993;21:59–69.

Holmes JC, Pruitt AL, Whalen NJ: Iliotibial band syndrome in cyclists. Am J Sports Med 1993;21:419–424.

Lebsack D, Gieck J, Saliba E: Iliotibial band friction syndrome. J Natl Athletic Trainer Assoc 1990;25:356–361.

Lucas CA: Iliotibial band friction syndrome as exhibited in athletes. J Natl Athletic Trainer Assoc 1992;27:250–252.

30

The Case of Postoperative Inflammation

A 64-year-old man with degenerative joint disease underwent a total knee replacement 6 weeks ago. He was seen for 10 days postoperatively as an inpatient and 3 times a week for 4 weeks as an outpatient while living with his daughter. You receive a home health referral to evaluate his progress and continue treatment.

Upon evaluation, you find the patient's range of motion for knee flexion is 70 degrees actively and 75 degrees passively; for knee extension the motion is –10 degrees actively and –5 degrees passively. The patient's strength is generally in the 4/5 range within available range of motion for the involved lower extremity. The patient's record indicates no increased range of motion over the past 2 weeks, but at end range of motion (flexion) pain is felt in the anterior distal thigh, 2 to 3 inches above the knee. The patient ambulates with one crutch inside and outside his home and says he walks frequently.

The patient's knee is slightly warm and edematous, and the patient states he commonly feels pain. The pain is greatest after therapy and typically lasts for 2 to 3 hours after each session. The patient states that when he performs his home exercise program (knee range of motion exercises and strengthening), his pain lasts for an hour or two.

What are your recommendations?

RESOLUTION

The cause of this patient's pain is an ongoing inflammatory response. The lack of range of motion made the therapist suspect that adhesions had developed as the result of chronic irritation. The chronic irritation had been excessive treatment during physical therapy and an overly aggressive exercise program. The patient had scar-tissue adhesions in the distal quadriceps muscles due to post-traumatic immobilization and chronic irritation.

The first step in this patient's treatment was to educate him in controlling his activity level and on the amount and intensity of exercise that he should perform. He was instructed to ambulate only within the house for the first 5 days, and to perform exercise in the pain-free range. That allowed the acute inflammation to subside. At the end of this period, range of motion improved approximately 5 degrees, and the pain diminished. The therapist then treated the adhesions with active exercises and passive stretching.

DISCUSSION

This case demonstrates the result of overly aggressive treatment protocols and a poorly monitored home exercise program. Critical factors were recognizing the excessive treatment and avoiding the threshold of stress that constituted the chronic irritation. The patient should have gained approximately 90 degrees of flexion 2 weeks after his operation. Proper initial treatment should have included appropriate repositioning during outpatient care to prevent the development of adhesions. That this patient initially had considerable pain for several hours after treatment and exercise indicates that the treatment approach was too aggressive. Pain following treatment and exercise should subside within 1 hour.

REFERENCES

Currier DP, Nelson RM (eds): *Dynamics of Human Biologic Tissues*. Philadelphia: Davis, 1992.

Kloth LC, McCulloch JM, Feeder JA (eds): *Wound Healing: Alternatives In Management*, second edition. Philadelphia: Davis, 1995.

Stanley BG, Tribuzi SM: *Concepts in Hand Rehabilitation*. Philadelphia: Davis, 1992.

31

The Case of Reflex Sympathetic Dystrophy

You receive a referral to evaluate a 34-year-old woman whose primary symptom is severe, burning pain in her right upper extremity. The pain has been present for approximately 10 weeks and has progressively worsened. The disorder has been diagnosed as reflex sympathetic dystrophy (RSD). The patient cannot relate any specific trauma or incident as the origin of pain. The patient's activities of daily living (ADLs) are impaired because of her reluctance to use the extremity. The patient is unable to perform any house cleaning, cooking, driving, or tasks that involve the use of her right upper extremity.

Upon evaluation, you find the skin of the patient's hand and forearm to be swollen, shiny, and red. The patient has hyperesthesia in the entire extremity. Active range of motion is limited in the shoulder, elbow, and wrist to approximately 75% of the uninvolved side, and finger range of motion is limited to 50% of the uninvolved side. You are unable to assess strength because of the pain. The patient does not attempt to use the arm at all and believes that if she rests the arm long enough it will get better by itself.

What are your recommendations?

RESOLUTION

This patient's belief that time would make her better and that if she continued to rest the arm the pain would decrease is contradictory to the typical management of RSD and may have increased the pain and left the patient less functional. The patient was treated with an approach that emphasized modalities, active exercise, and stress loading of the involved extremity.

A transcutaneous electrical nerve stimulation (TENS) unit was applied to the wrist and hand and provided good relief of pain. The patient performed active exercise 5 times a week. Part of the therapy included general conditioning exercises such as walking and swimming. Goal setting centered on self-selected objectives of increasing the patient's ability to perform ADLs, increasing endurance, and using the arm more frequently. Six weeks into the treatment program, the patient was able to resume some household activities, including occasional cooking for her family and house cleaning. Her tolerance for activity also improved.

DISCUSSION

RSD is a disorder characterized by chronic inflammation of one or more extremities. There are several theories about the mechanism behind the activity of the sympathetic nervous system in generating symptoms of RSD.

The first aspect of this patient's treatment was instructing her that if she wanted to re-cover, she was going to have to work toward it. In other words, initially the pain and swelling would probably increase. The concept that time would make it better had to be eliminated. The patient also was expected to resume some ADLs immediately as part of her treatment. A stress-loading program was initiated in which the patient was asked to scrub a hard surface three times a day for 10 minutes and to carry a purse containing 2 pounds in her hand throughout the day. The object of this stress-loading program was to provide neurovascular stress to and adaptation of the involved tissues. Pain-relieving modalities also were used as a part of the treatment plan.

It is important to recognize that patients with RSD typically do not recover fully within the course of physical therapy. Some have been known not to fully recover within the first year or two after onset. As such, continued monitoring and goal-setting by patients helps keep them actively working toward improving their condition.

REFERENCES

Levine D: Burning pain in an extremity: breaking the destructive cycle of reflex sympathetic dystrophy. Postgrad Med 1991;90:175–185.

Mandel S, Rothrock RW: Sympathetic dystrophies: recognizing and managing a puzzling group of syndromes. Postgrad Med 1990;87:213–218.

Watson HK, Carlson LK: Treatment of reflex sympathetic dystrophy of the hand with an active "stress loading" program. J Hand Surg 1987; 12:779–785.

32

The Case of Spinal Muscular Atrophy

Your patient is a 10-year-old girl with spinal muscular atrophy. She has severe proximal weakness but is able to perform household ambulation by keeping her shoulders posterior to her hip joints. The extreme lordotic posture gives her the stability she needs to compensate for poor abdominal and hip extensor strengths. The patient is scheduled to undergo spinal fusion with Harrington rod insertion in 3 weeks because of rapidly progressing scoliosis. You are concerned about the patient's ability to regain ambulation skills after the operation because the rigid alignment of the spine after fusion will not allow the lordotic posture.

How do you proceed?

RESOLUTION

The therapist decided the best approach was to contact the orthopedic surgeon to discuss concerns regarding the patient's return to ambulation. The therapist described her professional viewpoint: the child needed the mechanical advantage of alignment in excessive lordosis in order to balance standing and walking. The orthopedic surgeon agreed to consider this factor when performing the fusion. The surgeon contacted the therapist after the operation to tell the therapist some lordosis was retained during the fusion. The therapist saw the child after the operation and found that the patient retained enough lordosis to stand and walk.

DISCUSSION

Sometimes in the realities of a busy orthopedic surgical practice, physicians see patients in a different way than do physical therapists. The physician in this case was concerned with maximum correction of a rapidly progressing scoliosis. Her desired outcome was a rigid, straight spine. The physical therapist was concerned with functional ability after the operation. It was the balance between these two outlooks that benefited the patient the most.

REFERENCES

Cech D, Martio S: *Functional Movement Development Across the Life Span.* Philadelphia: Saunders, 1995.

Donatelli R: *The Biomechanics of the Foot and Ankle.* Philadelphia: Davis, 1990.

Tecklin JS (ed): *Pediatric Physical Therapy.* Philadelphia: Lippincott, 1989.

33

The Case of Changing the Environment

You are treating a 20-year-old woman who has cerebral palsy. She has been independent in wheelchair mobility, transfers to and from bed, and has required only minimum assistance with shower transfers. The last physical therapy she received was 7 years ago in the local school system. The therapy was discontinued when she changed schools.

The patient reports increased difficulty transferring from bed to wheelchair. The problem has become a barrier to independence. The patient sleeps in a water bed that contours to her postural contractures.

Treatment begins with extensive soft-tissue stretching to decrease hamstring, adductor, and hip flexor tightness. Inhibitory techniques are implemented to decrease spasticity, and positional mechanics are emphasized to increase the patient's ability to transfer out of bed.

Treatment proceeds for seven visits. The patient is discouraged because she remains unable to transfer out of bed independently. The patient reports that her other transfers (sit to stand, wheelchair to toilet, and wheelchair to chair) have become more difficult since therapy began.

How do you proceed?

RESOLUTION

The therapist recommended cutting the water bed box frame at the foot of the bed because that was where the patient performed her transfers. Soft-tissue stretching was discontinued because the patient's transfer ability had deteriorated with respect to all other transfers. Modifications to the bed improved the patient's ability to transfer out of bed. Discontinuing stretching allowed the patient to return to her previous level of soft-tissue contractures. Within 2 weeks the patient was independent in all transfers.

DISCUSSION

Patients with spastic disorders since childhood often learn to compensate for motor function and tasks. For various reasons, progression and deterioration in motor function occur in this population. Patients frequently use soft-tissue contractures to assist with stability during mobility. In this case, the stretching of soft-tissue contractures caused regression of transfer abilities. Discontinuing stretching allowed the functional contractures to return, and the patient's transfer ability returned to previous levels.

In some instances, however, changes to the physical environment facilitate self-reliant patient function. For this patient, the environment was a physical barrier. It was not the soft-tissue contractures that hampered functional mobility.

REFERENCES

Campbell SK: Efficacy of physical therapy in improving postural control in cerebral palsy. Pediatr Phys Ther 1990;2:135–140.

Campbell SK, Anderson J, Gardner HG: Physicians' beliefs in the efficacy of physical therapy in the management of cerebral palsy. Pediatr Phys Ther 1990;2:169–170.

Letts L, Law M, Rigby P, Cooper B, Stewart D, Strong S: Person-environment assessments in occupational therapy. Am J Occup Ther 1994; 48:608–618.

May BJ: *Home Health and Rehabilitation: Concepts of Care.* Philadelphia: Davis, 1993.

34

The Case of the Subacute Swollen Ankle

You have been asked to evaluate a 68-year-old woman who had undergone open reduction internal fixation of the left ankle 17 weeks ago. The injury was extremely traumatic, occurring as the patient missed a rung climbing down a ladder. The patient recounts her previous 6 weeks of physical therapy as unsuccessful. Treatment included moist heat, warm whirlpool, and active range of motion exercises. The patient discontinued treatment and pain medication and attempted self care at home for 5 weeks. During that time there were no improvements in pain, swelling, or ability to bear weight. The dysfunction has caused the patient to seek additional treatment.

Upon evaluation, you note the patient exhibits edema at the distal metatarsals, midfoot, and ankle. Range of motion is decreased compared with the other side at end ranges for all motions because of pain. The patient tolerates only toe-touch ambulation with bilateral axillary crutches.

How would you recommend treatment proceed?

RESOLUTION

The ankle complex includes synovial joints. Because of joint swelling, this patient's treatment consisted of compression wraps, cryotherapy, rest with elevation during non–weight-bearing periods, and emphasis on compliance with the physician's prescription for an anti-inflammatory medication. Weight-bearing was increased by progression to a single crutch then a cane; it concluded with independent ambulation as tolerated. After 6 weeks the patient's edema was 95% eliminated, range of motion was equal on bilateral comparison, and the patient was ambulating without assistive devices up to 3 hours per day.

DISCUSSION

The patient's original treatment program of warm whirlpool, moist heat, and range of motion exercises did not address the true nature of the problem. She reported the treatment felt good and that she could move her ankle well in the whirlpool, but she could not increase her tolerance to weight-bearing.

Even 17 weeks after the injury the importance of eliminating edema, the primary problem, from synovial joints remained a crucial element. The use of rest, ice, compression, elevation, and anti-inflammatory medication was clearly indicated.

Ice is used to reduce edema; compression and elevation aid venous return. Progressive weight-bearing assists in increasing bone density and the ability of soft tissue to endure mechanical stresses. Elimination of edema is, of course, the primary consideration for all pathologic conditions that involve a synovial joint.

REFERENCES

Eiff MP, Smith AT, Smith GE: Early mobilization versus immobilization in the treatment of lateral ankle sprains. Am J Sports Med 1994;22:83–88.

Mascaro TB, Swanson LE: Rehabilitation of the foot and ankle. Orthop Clin North Am 1994;25:147–160.

Trevino SS, Davis P, Hecht PJ: Management of acute and chronic lateral ligament injuries of the ankle. Orthop Clin North Am 1994;25:1–16.

Wilkerson GB, Nitz AJ: Dynamic ankle stability: mechanical and neuromuscular interrelationships. J Sport Rehabil 1994;3:43–57.

35

The Case of the Myocardial Infarction

You are requested to evaluate a 57-year-old man who was origi-
nally admitted to the hospital with cardiogenic shock after suffering a myocardial infarction. His past medical history
includes ischemic cardiomyopathy, myocardial infarctions in
1987, 1990, and 1992, hypertension, and recurrent congestive
heart failure that began in 1992. Because of hemodynamic instability, the patient spent approximately 2 months in the intensive
care unit and needed a tracheotomy for prolonged ventilator
dependency. While in the intensive care unit the patient could
tolerate only passive to active-assisted range of motion. Dobutamine has been prescribed to increase the patient's cardiac
output.

For 3 weeks you have treated this patient for deficits in functional mobility, decreased strength, and decreased cardiopulmonary and musculoskeletal endurance. The patient requires
minimal assistance of one for bed mobility and maximal assistance of one for transfers. He tolerates approximately 45 seconds of continuous activity before demonstrating shortness of
breath and muscular fatigue.

Over the next 3 weeks there is a gradual increase in strength
and functional mobility followed by a decline, resulting in a decrease in exercise tolerance. As a result of the patient's decline,
you begin to question whether rehabilitation is feasible.

What is your recommendation?

RESOLUTION

The primary problem was that the patient's therapy was not progressing. After a thorough review of the case, the therapist recognized that the episodes of exercise intolerance corresponded with decreases in dosage of the inotropic medication Dobutamine. The therapist consulted the physician to coordinate care plans. The physician prescribed a level of dobutamine that allowed progress in physical therapy.

DISCUSSION

This patient had ischemic cardiomyopathy. The problems presented were the result of coronary artery disease and repeated myocardial infarctions. The infarctions impaired the ability of the myocardium to contract and maintain cardiac output. Cardiac output is the amount of blood ejected from the heart each minute.

This patient could not tolerate progression in functional mobility because his heart could not increase cardiac output as workload increased. Dobutamine is a commonly used medication for patients with cardiomyopathy. This drug has a positive inotropic effect that directly stimulates the beta receptors in the heart to increase the force of myocardial contraction. With the increase in contractility, the ability of the heart to maintain cardiac output improves.

This case demonstrates the importance of coordinating services among the health care team. To help restore patients to the highest level of function, therapists must be aware of the medical management plan. Modifying the inotropic medication to align the dosage with the goals of physical therapy enabled the patient to increase his exercise tolerance and level of functional mobility. When his strength and exercise tolerance improved, the patient was slowly weaned from the dobutamine. At the time of discharge from the hospital, the patient tolerated approximately 1 hour of continuous physical therapy and was weaned successfully from the dobutamine. After a 4-week stay in an inpatient rehabilitation hospital, the patient returned home functionally independent.

REFERENCES

Ciccone CD: *Pharmacology in Rehabilitation*. Philadelphia: Davis, 1990.

Clouchesy JM, Brev C, Cardin S, Rudy, EB, Whittaker AA: *Critical Care Nursing*. Philadelphia: Saunders, 1993.

Dennison RD: Understanding the four determinants of cardiac output. Nursing 1990;20:34–42.

Frownfelter DL (ed): *Chest Physical Therapy and Pulmonary Rehabilitation: An Interdisciplinary Approach*, second edition. St. Louis: Mosby Year Book, 1987.

Hillegass EA, Sadowsky HS: *Essentials of Cardiopulmonary Physical Therapy*. Philadelphia: Saunders, 1994.

36

The Case of Shortness of Breath

The patient is a 78-year-old woman who recently sustained a cerebral vascular accident that resulted in moderate muscular weakness in the right upper and lower extremities. Her daughter reports the patient has been taking digoxin, quinidine, and furosemide. During the last week, however, the daughter has noted a decrease in the patient's ability to complete activities of daily living without assistance. The daughter is becoming increasingly concerned about the amount of care her mother requires. You are requested to evaluate the patient in her home.

Upon evaluation, the patient reports shortness of breath. She also reports that she is frequently disrupted from sleep with a sense of being short of breath. The patient indicates that she feels more comfortable sleeping in a recliner chair. You palpate an irregular heart rate of 100 to 120 beats per minute and pitting edema in both lower extremities.

When ascertaining her physical capabilities you notice that the patient requires minimal assistance of one for transfers and walks with a wide-base quad cane. She reports dizziness when she is in an upright standing posture, which further interferes with mobility. You determine that the patient's blood pressure drops with changes in posture.

What is your recommendation?

RESOLUTION

Two primary problems were identified in this case. First, the therapist was concerned about the patient's decrease in exercise tolerance, increase in shortness of breath and peripheral edema, and the high, irregular heart rate. The therapist referred the patient back to the family physician for management of possible congestive heart failure and control of heart rate and rhythm.

The second problem was the orthostatic hypotension that occurred when the patient changed postures. This may have been related to the abnormally high heart rate and to the fact that the patient had been essentially immobile because of recent hospital admissions. The orthostatic hypotension also was related to the patient's deconditioning.

Once cardiac status was under control, the therapist had the patient use support stockings or elastic wraps. The patient also was asked to perform lower extremity isotonic exercise and gradually institute isometric activities for the lower extremities before moving into an upright posture. These treatment strategies increased venous return and allowed for an increase in the patient's tolerance for upright activity.

Remaining aware of the signs and symptoms of congestive heart failure and an irregular heart rate may prevent further hospitalization or a decline in functional mobility. In this case, after medications were changed, the patient was able to address the problems of orthostatic hypotension caused by deconditioning. The patient's and therapist's efforts resulted in the patient's regaining an independent functional mobility level in her home.

DISCUSSION

It is not uncommon for a physical therapist providing home health care to observe a deterioration in a patient's medical condition. In this case, the patient had signs of congestive heart failure. The peripheral edema was the result of a decrease in the ability of the heart to pump an adequate amount of blood. In response to a decrease in circulating volume, the kidneys respond by decreasing the amount of fluid excreted. This excess fluid is then displaced in the extracellular spaces of the body, such as the lower extremities, sacrum, and abdomen. Therapists should document the severity of peripheral edema by obtaining girth measurements, monitoring weight gain, or rating the degree of pitting edema.

This patient also demonstrated a decrease in exercise capacity with an increase in shortness of breath. She described having paroxysmal nocturnal dyspnea, which is commonly the result of fluid accumulation in the lungs, particularly when a patient is supine. The patient also described orthopnea, which is the sense of being short of breath in a recumbent position. The patient described being more comfortable sleeping in a recliner chair. In this position the fluid may be more likely to drain from the lungs.

An irregular heart rate is a clinical sign of a dysrhythmia, in this case atrial fibrillation. At greater than 100 to 120 beats per minute at rest, heart rate is considered uncontrolled. At such an elevated rate, the decrease in cardiac output may cause patients to report feeling slightly dizzy or light-headed. The medications the patient was taking, digoxin and quinidine, are commonly used by patients with a history of congestive heart failure and atrial fibrillation. Quinidine suppresses the excessive heart rate, and digoxin increases the contractility of the heart and decreases heart rate.

REFERENCES

Ciccone CD: *Pharmacology in Rehabilitation*. Philadelphia: Davis, 1990.

Clouchesy JM, Brev C, Cardin S, Rudy, EB, Whittaker AA: *Critical Care Nursing*. Philadelphia: Saunders, 1993.

Dennison RD: Understanding the four determinants of cardiac output. Nursing 1990;20:34–42.

Hillegass EA, Sadowsky HS: *Essentials of Cardiopulmonary Physical Therapy*. Philadelphia: Saunders, 1994.

Irwin S, Techlin JS (eds): *Cardiopulmonary Physical Therapy*, second edition. St. Louis: Mosby, 1990.

37

The Case of Emphysema

You receive a consultation for functional retraining and strengthening for a 54-year-old man with end-stage lung disease secondary to emphysema. The patient reports that he can walk only 10 feet because of weakness and dyspnea and that he requires assistance with all activities of daily living. During the evaluation you document that the patient desaturates on 4 L of oxygen. He particularly desaturates with activities that involve his upper extremities and standing, even with 6 L of oxygen. There is little diaphragmatic movement, a finding confirmed with a radiographic report that notes a flattened position.

What are your recommendations?

RESOLUTION

The primary problems were the patient's level of deconditioning and functional impairment. These problems were directly related to pulmonary disease and the level of dyspnea. The therapist determined that the patient did not desaturate in a supported, seated position. The patient also had increased exercise tolerance when he used his lower extremities in a supported position. Therefore, the best approach was to design a rehabilitation program for cardiopulmonary reconditioning and strengthening in a semi-reclined posture. After this treatment, the patient was discharged from the hospital ambulating more than 150 feet with a wheeled walker and comfortably tolerating 15 minutes of interval cardiopulmonary reconditioning. The program consisted of interval training on a pedal exerciser and general therapeutic strengthening exercises. The patient was given a breathing exercise program to strengthen his accessory respiratory muscles.

DISCUSSION

Designing a rehabilitation program that focuses on an appropriate patient position allows the patient to begin cardiopulmonary endurance training and strengthening. In a reclined position the trunk and upper extremities are stabilized on a supporting structure. This allows the accessory respiratory muscles (pectoralis major, pectoralis minor, and serratus anterior) to reverse their muscle action and assist in inspiration. In a trunk-supported position, the abdominal muscles also become accessory expiratory muscles.

Because the patient's diaphragm did not function properly, training accessory respiratory muscles was important. From a flattened position the diaphragm loses its proper length-tension relationship and can no longer effectively support ventilatory needs. During inspiration, the upper ribs move in a superior and anterior direction while the lower rib cage moves superiorly and laterally. This motion is a result of rotation and gliding at the costovertebral and costotransverse joints and slight extension of the thoracic spine.

A therapist who knows the kinematics of the thorax can help a patient increase respiratory efficiency by coordinating the breathing pattern with gross motor activities. Activities that require a patient to reach overhead should be accompanied by inspiration and trunk flexion. Reaching downward should be accompanied by expiration.

A nontraditional cardiopulmonary rehabilitation approach was necessary to help this patient benefit from an exercise program. Results included an increase in endurance, reflecting improved cardiovascular and musculoskeletal efficiency to perform work. Heart rate decreased and peripheral circulation improved after training. These improvements resulted in an increase in functional mobility within the limits of the pulmonary disease. Because he needed to use accessory respiratory muscles to increase his upright functional mobility, the patient was given a four-wheeled walker. The four-wheeled walker decreased the energy the patient needed to ambulate within his environment and provided continuous stabilization of the upper extremities and trunk. The stabilization resulted in an increased efficiency in his breathing pattern.

REFERENCES

Frownfelter DL (ed): *Chest Physical Therapy and Pulmonary Rehabilitation: An Interdisciplinary Approach*, second edition. St. Louis: Mosby Year Book, 1987.

Hillegass EA, Sadowsky HS: *Essentials of Cardiopulmonary Physical Therapy*. Philadelphia: Saunders, 1994.

Irwin S, Techlin JS (eds): *Cardiopulmonary Physical Therapy*, second edition. St. Louis: Mosby Year Book, 1990.

38

The Case of the Gunshot Wound

You receive a referral to evaluate a 28-year-old man admitted to the hospital after suffering a gunshot wound to the chest. The patient underwent repair of the right ventricle and partial right pneumonectomy. He required full cardiopulmonary support with extracorporeal membrane oxygenation (ECMO) because of the severity of his hemodynamic instability. Until postoperative day 26, physical therapy goals included maintaining range of motion and prevention of pressure ulcers. ECMO was discontinued on postoperative day 28, and the patient began to participate in therapy. Over the next week you notice a continuous decrease in the range of motion in both knees. The thighs are warm, painful, and swollen. There is a hard end-feel to the knee joints.

What are your recommendations?

RESOLUTION

The first step was to notify a cardiothoracic critical care physician regarding the regression of lower extremity function. An initial impression was that heterotrophic ossification (HO) was developing. HO is the formation of mature trabecular bone along the connecting tissue between muscle planes. Magnetic resonance images showed developing bilateral immature HO at the distal femoral and proximal tibial regions. The patient was given diphosphate, which inhibits bone metabolism and has been found effective in the management of immature HO.

The physical therapy plan for the lower extremities consisted of gentle range of motion within tolerance and tissue restrictions (aggressive range of motion and manipulation are thought to contribute to the progressive development of HO). Grade one and two joint mobilizations were performed at the patellofemoral, tibiofibular, and tibiofemoral joints. Because this patient was able to assist in his physical therapy program, contract-hold techniques were used to increase range of motion.

Special care was taken to address the cardiopulmonary trauma. The patient began cardiopulmonary reconditioning by using an upper extremity ergometer. Postural drainage positions were used to promote pulmonary hygiene and were incorporated into a general therapeutic exercise routine for strengthening. Breathing exercises, techniques to release the soft tissue of the intercostal spaces, and joint mobilization were used to increase chest wall expansion. Once lower extremity strength and range of motion improved, gait training was initiated with use of a walker. Range of motion and strength were progressed with isokinetic exercise and a stationary bicycle.

DISCUSSION

The incidence of HO is highly variable. It occurs in 40% of patients with spinal cord injuries and 10% to 15% of patients with head injuries. HO occurs in 50% of patients with total hip replacements, 30% to 50% of whom have clinical limitations in range of motion of the hip joint. HO also has been reported in patients who sustain burns severe enough to require hospitalization and patients with prolonged pharmacologically induced coma.

The earliest manifestations of HO include localized edema, pain, and loss of range of motion. These findings may be mistaken for deep vein thrombosis, cellulitis, acute arthritis, or intramuscular bleeding. Serum calcium and phosphate levels are usually within normal limits, but the serum alkaline phosphate level is elevated during the active osteogenesis phase.

As a result of quick problem recognition, this patient's condition was diagnosed early and managed appropriately. The patient advanced to independence with transfers, ambulation, and stair climbing with a straight cane. Bilateral knee flexion increased to 90 degrees, and the patient was discharged home to continue physical therapy on an outpatient basis.

REFERENCES

Clements NC, Camilli AE: Heterotopic ossification complicating critical illness. Chest 1993;104:1526–1528.

Frownfelter DL (ed): Chest Physical Therapy and Pulmonary Rehabilitation: An Interdisciplinary Approach, second edition. St. Louis: Mosby Year Book, 1987.

Hillegass EA, Sadowsky HS: Essentials of Cardiopulmonary Physical Therapy. Philadelphia: Saunders, 1994.

Irwin S, Techlin JS (eds): Cardiopulmonary Physical Therapy, second edition. St. Louis: Mosby Year Book, 1990.

Sawyer JR, Myers MA, Rosier RN, Puzas JE: Heterotopic ossification: clinical and cellular aspects. Calcif Tissue Int 1991;49:208–215.

Voss DE, Ionta MK, Myers BT: Proprioceptive Neuromuscular Facilitation, third edition. Philadelphia: Harper & Row, 1985.

39

The Case of Bell's Palsy

The patient is a 32-year-old man who is otherwise healthy. Two weeks ago, when he awakened in the morning, he noticed a drooping of the right corner of his mouth and an inability to completely close the right eye. Later that day, he visited his physician, who made a diagnosis of Bell's palsy. The physician prescribed oral corticosteriods for 1 week (the medications were gradually discontinued during the second week) and use of an eye patch and referred the patient for physical therapy.

On the first day of physical therapy treatment (1 day after onset of the palsy), the patient is unable to voluntarily contract any of the muscles innervated by the right seventh cranial nerve. You produce strong twitch and sustained contractions with a high-voltage pulsed-current stimulator. The stimulation parameters are as follows: monophasic pulses at a 20 microsec phase duration and 30 Hz at an amplitude set to produce strong contractions (110 V on the first day of treatment). The stimulation is delivered with a monopolar electrode system. You use a 1-cm diameter hand-held electrode (cathode) to apply current to the seventh cranial nerve and the involved muscles, and a 10-cm by 10-cm dispersive electrode (anode) was fastened to the right arm.

Each day, you need to increase the amplitude of stimulation to produce contractions as strong as those of the previous day. By the 14th day of treatment, you can produce contractions that are only barely visible even with the amplitude set to the machine maximum (500 V). Paralysis of the facial musculature on the right side persists.

Can you do anything else to produce strong contractions?

RESOLUTION

The therapist determined the chronaxie value for the affected muscles so the appropriate pulse duration for treatment could be selected. A stimulator that can produce pulses of long duration (10 msec) or one with continuous-flow low-voltage direct current was required. Amplitude was set high enough to produce vigorous muscle contractions. When pulses were used, a rate from 10 Hz to 25 Hz was found most beneficial. Subsequent stimulation treatments were given three times a day, including three sets of 20 isometric contractions. The therapist observed for, and avoided, fatigue by allowing at least 5 seconds of rest between contractions and 1 minute of rest between sets. Muscular atrophy was delayed, and as reinnervation occurred the patient made a full recovery.

DISCUSSION

Wallerian degeneration appears to have caused the denervation of muscles innervated by the seventh cranial nerve. This theory is supported by the continued paralysis of muscle and an inability to produce contractions with wave forms of short pulse duration. The pulse duration being used (20 microsec) was too short to depolarize denervated muscle. As the Wallerian degeneration proceeded and progressively fewer muscle fibers remained innervated, it became more and more difficult to produce a visible contraction with short-duration pulses.

The appropriate use of electrical stimulation can delay muscle fiber degeneration and shorten recovery time. Because denervated muscle has a great capacity to store electrical charge, the stimulation device used must produce a long-duration (greater than 10 msec) monophasic wave form to create an action potential (and contraction). High-voltage pulsed-current stimulators are not capable of producing the pulse duration required to depolarize denervated muscle.

Electrophysiologic testing can help clarify prognosis and guide treatment. Increased latencies with nerve conduction velocity testing can indicate denervation. In this case the normal range for latencies to triangularis, frontalis, and orbicularis oris muscles was 3.5 to 5.0 msec. If a muscle response can be produced, and the latencies are within normal range, the prognosis for recovery is often very good.

Peripheral axons regenerate at the rate of 1 to 2 mm per day. The distance from the point of entrapment (petrous portion of temporal bone) to the most distal muscle affected should be measured so expected reinnervation time can be calculated. It is generally recommended that stimulation be continued for a period of 4 to 6 weeks after reinnervation occurs.

REFERENCES

Bannister R: *Brain's Clinical Neurology,* third edition. Cary, NC: Oxford University Press, 1969.

Chusid JG: *Correlative Neuroanatomy and Functional Neurology,* sixteenth edition. Los Altos: Lange, 1976.

Downey JA, Myers SJ, Gonzalez EG, Lieberman JS (eds): *The Physiological Basis of Rehabilitation,* second edition. Boston: Butterworth-Heinemann, 1994.

Echternach JL: *Introduction to Electromyography and Nerve Conduction Testing: A Laboratory Manual.* Thorofare: Slack, 1994.

Gersh MR (ed): *Electrotherapy in Rehabilitation.* Philadelphia: Davis, 1992.

Nelson RM, Currier DP: *Clinical Electrotherapy,* second edition. East Norwalk: Appleton & Lange, 1991.

40

The Case of the 4-month-old Baby

You are requested to perform an initial evaluation of a 4-month-old baby referred to physical therapy for developmental stimulation because of severe global hypotonia and developmental delay. Her neonatal history includes the surgical removal of the upper lobe of the right lung 5 days after birth because of cystic malformation. There have been no postsurgical complications, but the baby has not developed head control and movement patterns typical of a 4-month-old baby.

As you begin the evaluation, the mother warns you that the baby is still sensitive around the right chest area and does not tolerate lying on her right side. The mother describes the infant as a perfectly content baby, except during sudden episodes of distress when the baby cries because of apparent pain and fatigue. The mother also tells you these symptoms are related to colic. The mother tells you the episodes of distress and crying have been increasing in frequency and are more likely to occur when the baby is relaxed or asleep.

While observing the infant, you note she is a quietly alert and smiling baby who exhibits limited spontaneous movement, except for intermittent pelvic elevation on the left. The baby maintains an asymmetric posture while lying on her back. The mother indicates that this is her preferred posture. You notice that the lower portion of the sternum is slightly indented and that considerable flaring of the lower ribs is present, the right ribs being somewhat elevated.

To ascertain trunk symmetry, you begin to test the infant's tolerance to alignment and movement facilitation, especially around the area described by the mother as sensitive. To your surprise the baby tolerates your evaluation and handling extremely well. There is no apparent tenderness to touch or movement of the tissues and structures surrounding the surgical scar. This is also true in the area along the inner and lower borders of the right scapula.

Passive ranging of the right shoulder girdle and rib cage is tolerated in all directions. Side-lying posture on the right is attained with minimal discomfort, but the baby immediately drops back into her preferred asymmetric supine position. As you start to align the pelvis into midline, the ribs gradually move into a retraction motion that appears to be much stronger on the right than on the left. The sternum sinks deeper into the chest, and a breathing pattern of short breaths quickly develops. The infant emits a strained cry, and the mother reports that the baby is beginning to experience colic. By observing the inward pulling of the ribs and sternum and by the sound of the cry, you realize that there is more to this than simply colic.

What is the cause of this episode and how can you help alleviate the problem?

RESOLUTION

The therapist placed her fingers 1 inch below the base of the baby's sternum, putting light pressure on the abdominal cavity while gently pulling down on the muscles and soft tissue toward the pelvis. This maneuver released the diaphragm. The therapist repeated this procedure two or three times until a normal breathing pattern was restored, and the child stopped crying. The therapist taught the technique to the mother so she could assist the child when episodes occurred at home. The frequency of episodes was reduced by 90% within 4 to 5 weeks. Acquisition of developmental skills became much easier to facilitate as a result of the improvement in head and trunk control.

DISCUSSION

It is unusual for colic to persist beyond the first 3 months of life, especially in babies who are not very active. The diaphragm is the primary muscle of respiration, but children with muscular dysfunction often use it for fixing the trunk when postural control is reduced or missing. The mechanical balance of this infant's rib-cage mobility was influenced by hypotonicity and postsurgical asymmetry. The upper lobe is the largest of the three lobes of the right lung. When the lobe is removed, the two lower lobes expand and move upward to fill the available thoracic space. In this infant, the right side of the diaphragm followed the same upward direction.

To counteract the asymmetric pull, the child compensated by elevating the opposite side of the pelvis. The left quadratus lumborum muscle, which assists the diaphragm in respiration by connecting the pelvis with the lower ribs, was activated. This contributed to postural fixation. The reluctance of the child to lie on her right side was not because of increased sensitivity but because of an attempt to preserve this fixation. When passive alignment was performed, or when the infant was relaxed or asleep, the fixation was occasionally lost, causing the diaphragm to contract and to pull upward. A hypotonic child who lies primarily supine may need to work hard to ventilate because the abdominal viscera impede the full descent of the diaphragm. By helping the child attain other postures, trunk control improves, and the diaphragm can return to its primary function of respiration.

REFERENCES

Boehmi R: Assessment and treatment of the respiratory system for breathing, sound production and trunk control. Teamtalk 1992;2:2–8.

Shelov SP, Hannemann RE (eds): *The American Academy of Pediatrics: Caring for Your Baby and Young Child, Birth to Age 5.* New York: Bantam, 1993.

Shidlow DV, Smith DS: *A Practical Guide to Pediatric Respiratory Diseases.* Philadelphia: Hanley & Belfus, 1994.

Tecklin JS (ed): *Pediatric Physical Therapy,* second edition. Philadelphia: Lippincott, 1994.

41

The Case of Severe Torticollis

You receive a referral for evaluation and treatment of a 7-year-old girl who suffered a left clavicular fracture and severe right torticollis. The injury occurred when the child was accidentally thrown from a seesaw at a playground. The patient was hospitalized for a week for treatment of cervical spasms and fracture stabilization. During the last 2 days at the hospital, the patient was placed in horizontal cervical traction using small amounts of weight (2 to 3 pounds) for as long as 3 hours as tolerated. The patient showed gradual improvement and was sent home yesterday with a muscle relaxant and pain medication to be administered only when needed. The physician requested that traction be continued at home, and a home health nurse was assigned to monitor both the medication and the traction unit.

Because no home health physical therapist was available, the child has been referred to your outpatient facility for daily treatments. A radiology report indicates proper healing at the fracture site and no vertebral fractures.

When you evaluate her, the child reports increased pain with areas of tenderness both on the torticollis side and on the back of the neck. You notice the child does not present a typical torticollis posture, in which the chin is rotated away from the side of the shortened muscle with the head tilted toward the side of the shortening. Instead, the chin is rotated toward the restricted right side with the shoulder of the restricted side elevated toward the chin. The head is displaced slightly backward and toward the left. The mother reports this posture becomes more prominent when the child experiences pain and stiffness or during periods of prolonged sitting or standing.

You proceed with a treatment of moist heat, followed by gentle soft-tissue stretching and muscle relaxation techniques performed with the patient in the supine posture. The child attains considerable pain relief, gaining 15 to 20 degrees of active neck rotation toward midline and relaxing the right shoulder down by 1 to 2 inches.

When she returns for treatment, the child appears to be in excruciating pain. The mother comments that the motion obtained during therapy did not last for more than 1 hour. Afterward there was continuous pain that required medication. As a result, the child poorly tolerated traction for a period of 1 to 2 hours.

How do you proceed?

RESOLUTION

The therapist wondered if the home traction unit was functioning properly and arranged for a home visit after the treatment session. The unit was properly installed at the child's bed, and the mother demonstrated the correct way to fit the harness on the child. After 3 to 4 minutes the child began to tilt her head backward and toward the left in response to mild spasm. She was able to realign herself well, but a few minutes later the same reaction occurred, this time causing a defense reaction on the torticollis side. The muscles contracted, and the shoulder began elevating once again. The therapist realized that the traction was not providing the therapeutic effect needed.

The therapist responded to the problem by calling the physician. After a brief discussion they agreed on a 2- to 3-day trial period without traction and substituted use of a soft cervical collar. Treatment during this period focused on relaxation of the upper trapezius muscle.

The patient experienced gradual improvement over the next 3 days. The use of pain medication was reduced by 50%. The physician agreed to extend the time off traction for another week, and the child began to acquire active control of the neck muscles. The pain appeared only after the child spent 2 to 3 hours sitting or standing, indicating the possibility that vertebral compression existed during upright postures. Traction treatments were re-started, and the child demonstrated steady improvement. Eventually pain medication was no longer needed, and the torticollis was fully resolved within 6 weeks.

DISCUSSION

Traction is effective in alleviating pressure on nerve roots affected by compression of the vertebrae. For cervical traction to be effective, 25 to 30 degrees of midline cervical flexion needs to be maintained to obtain desirable distraction of the cervical spine. Because the child's torticollis involved a strong rotation component toward the shortened side, this alignment was difficult to attain consistently. When the left upper trapezius went into spasm, an extra strain was imposed on the already tight cervical muscles on the right. This began a cycle of pain and increased stiffness on the torticollis side. Once the left upper trapezius was completely relaxed, it was easier to release the right side of the neck. This allowed proper cervical flexion, and the patient received maximum benefit from traction treatment.

REFERENCES

Brewer K: Identifying and treating torticollis. Clin Manage 1990; 10:19–21.

Emery C: The determinants of treatment duration for congenital muscular torticollis. Phys Ther 1994;74:921–929.

Grieve GP: *Modern Manual Therapy of the Vertebral Column*. New York: Churchill Livingstone, 1986.

Kerrick RC, French C: Torticollis: a head and neck immobilizer. Am J Occup Ther 1993;47:79–80.

Nypaber M, Treloar D: Neutral cervical spine positioning in children. Ann Emerg Med 1994;23:208–211.

Perrin JCS, Badell A, Binder H, Dystra DD, Easton JKM, Matthews DJ, et al: Pediatric rehabilitation. Musculoskeletal and soft tissue disorders part 6. Arch Phys Med Rehab 1989;70:183–189.

Saunders HD, Saunders R: *Evaluation, Treatment and Prevention of Musculoskeletal Disorders*. Minneapolis: Viking, 1985.

42

The Case of the Weak Spell

You are a home health care physical therapist. For the past 3 weeks you have been treating a 68-year-old woman who was discharged from an acute care hospital. Her history includes being taken to the hospital emergency department by ambulance after suffering a weak spell at home. When emergency medical services responded to the patient's home they found her to have dyspnea, swollen ankles and feet, jugular vein distention, rales through both lung fields, and a rapid pulse. The patient required immediate oxygen.

Additional information obtained in the emergency department included a history of a gastric ulcer and fluid retention in both lower extremities. Further examination and testing confirmed a diagnosis of congestive heart failure. The patient was given a number of medications designed to assist with her medical condition, including a diuretic. Her condition dramatically improved during the next 24 hours. The patient was discharged from the hospital 1 week after admission.

Because she had limited strength and endurance, the patient was referred to physical therapy for evaluation and treatment. The initial evaluation revealed 3/5 muscle strength in the major muscle groups of the upper and lower extremities. Home health therapy has greatly increased her strength and endurance. Today, however, the patient indicates she is having a bad day, and you note that she is responding inappropriately to questions. It appears as if the swelling has returned to the lower extremities.

What action do you take?

RESOLUTION

The patient had a history of a gastric ulcer. To alleviate the gastric discomfort she encountered while taking prescribed medications, the patient had also been taking an over-the-counter (OTC) antacid. The therapist suspected the OTC drug may have reduced the effectiveness of one of the prescribed medications. The patient was transferred to the hospital for additional examination and testing.

The emergency department physician ordered immediate blood tests that confirmed the therapist's suspicion. Tests indicated the OTC medication had reduced the effectiveness of the congestive heart failure medication. Once the OTC medication was discontinued, the patient's signs and symptoms cleared, and she returned home 48 hours later. The patient was followed in home care physical therapy for 2 more weeks and then discharged having met all goals.

DISCUSSION

Knowledge of medication interaction is important for therapists involved in home care physical therapy. When blood chemistry levels do not fall within normal ranges, there may be a rapid deterioration in a patient's mental and physical status. The patient in this case presented physical and mental changes that occurred in a very short period of time. This lead the therapist to suspect a medication-related problem.

REFERENCES

Ciccone CD: *Pharmacology in Rehabilitation*. Philadelphia: Davis, 1990.

Eddy L: *Physical Therapy Pharmacology*. St. Louis: Mosby, 1992.

Hillegass EA, Sadowsky HS: *Essentials of Cardiopulmonary Physical Therapy*. Philadelphia: Saunders, 1994.

Kessler CM: The pharmacology of aspirin, heparin, coumarin, and thrombolytic agents: implications for therapeutic use in cardiopulmonary disease 1991;99:97s–112s.

43

The Case of the Ankle Ulcer

You are a consultant to a number of facilities, including a local nursing home. From that home comes a call from the director of nursing regarding a patient's nonhealing wound, which has worsened since admission. The patient is a 60-year-old woman who has resided at the nursing home for 2 weeks. Before her admission, the patient was hospitalized briefly to begin wound care. The wound is a result of blunt trauma sustained while the patient lived in her own apartment.

Your careful questioning reveals that the patient had a venous stasis ulcer in the same location several years ago. The ulcer healed successfully with conservative treatment. The patient was previously independent in all activities of daily living. The goal on admission to the nursing home was to return the patient to her previous home and lifestyle.

You evaluate the patient and find her confused and unable to clearly answer your questions. An aide reports that the patient is no longer transferring with assistance of one and must be lifted. The patient now requires assistance to eat. The nursing staff reports that because the patient reported pain during dressing changes, a physician prescribed a narcotic pain medication.

You carefully soak and remove the dressing, noticing an 8 cm x 6 cm draining wound on the medial side of the left ankle. The wound bed appears beefy red and has several small areas of active bleeding. The surrounding skin is macerated and pigmented, and the area is slightly edematous. The current treatment is povidone-iodine wet-to-dry dressings, changed each shift. The director of nursing is concerned that the patient may not return home and asks if you can assist in the plan of care.

What are your recommendations?

RESOLUTION

The problem in this case was the method of wound care. Wet-to-dry dressings are a nonselective form of debridement and can remove granulation tissue when they are changed. Removal of granulation tissue impairs wound healing. The pain caused by this method of wound care required relief with a narcotic analgesic. Narcotics can cause changes in cognition, including confusion. The therapist recommended discontinuation of the wet-to-dry dressings and use of a dressing suitable to a draining wound. In this case, a calcium alginate dressing was selected to manage the drainage, reduce skin maceration, promote healing, and eliminate the need for pain medication.

DISCUSSION

This case outlines the tendency of some facilities to treat wounds ineffectively. Modern wound care emphasizes a moist wound environment, something a wet-to-dry dressing violates. Allowing the wound to dry impairs wound healing. Some solutions used as part of a wet-to-dry dressing may impair wound healing because the clinical concentrations are cytotoxic to fibroblasts and myofibroblasts.

Wet-to-dry dressings can be very painful when removed. Some caregivers may be tempted to use a whirlpool to facilitate dressing removal and wound cleaning. Although hydrotherapy may make dressing removal easier, a whirlpool with even moderate agitation may damage vulnerable endothelial cells. Those cells are best treated by protecting them with an appropriate dressing.

The dressing selected was a calcium alginate product. Alginate dressings absorb drainage, reduce bleeding and skin maceration, and reduce or eliminate pain at the time of dressing change. Because they are saline-soluble, the dressing and exudate are simply flushed from the area with sterile saline solution. Because the dressing is saline-soluble, not water-soluble, hydrotherapy would be ineffective in removing a calcium alginate dressing.

When the appropriate dressing was used, the patient no longer required pain medication. Within 2 days the patient's confusion was eliminated, and the patient fully participated in her care. One week later she was discharged to her own home with follow-up care provided by a home health agency. The wound subsequently healed and the patient remained independent in community living.

REFERENCES

Andrews LW: The perils of povidone-iodine use. Ostomy Wound Manage 1994;40:68,70,72–73.

Ciccone CD: *Pharmacology in Rehabilitation*. Philadelphia: Davis, 1990.

Foresman PA, Payne DS, Becker D, Lewis D, Rodeheaver GT: Wounds: a compendium of clinical research and practice. Wounds 1993;5:226–231.

Fowler EV: Equipment and products used in management and treatment of pressure ulcers. Nurs Clin North Am 1987;22:449–461.

Gensheimer D: A review of calcium alginates. Ostomy Wound Manage 1993;39:34–43.

Kloth LC, McCulloch JM, Feeder JA: *Wound Healing: Alternatives in Management*, second edition. Philadelphia: Davis, 1995.

Moran M, Brimer M: Sorbsan: a topical wound care dressing—a literature review and implications for physical therapists. Geri-Topics 1992;15:15–19.

Rodeheaver G, Bellamy W, Kody M, Spatafora G: Bactericidal activity and toxicity of iodine containing solutions in wounds. Arch Surg 1982;117:181–185.

Smith LH: Povidone-iodine: potential adverse reactions. Oncol Nurs Forum 1991;18:134.

Welch JS: Efficiency and safety of povidone-iodine underscored. J Emerg Nurs 1992;18:191–192.

44

The Case of Orthopedic Fatigue

You are a staff physical therapist in a skilled nursing facility. The patient is a 59-year-old woman with a history of interstitial pulmonary fibrosis. She was admitted to the facility after an open reduction internal fixation of the right hip because of a fracture. The hip repair was performed 8 days ago. From a chart review you learn the patient had been independent in self care but required assistance with grocery shopping, heavy cleaning, and other home activities. The report received from the hospital indicates the patient tired quickly and was barely able to transfer to a bedside commode. She was able to ambulate only 5 feet with a walker bearing partial weight on the right lower extremity. The patient had to stop ambulating because of fatigue and shortness of breath.

During the initial evaluation you find the patient is pale but not cyanotic. When she sits the patient's heart rate is 120 beats per minute, blood pressure is 100/80 mmHg, and respirations are 34 per minute. The patient's strength, range of motion, sensation, and balance are all normal or at least sufficient for ambulation with a walker. During the first 2 to 3 days in the skilled nursing facility, the patient has been unable to progress beyond the level described in the hospital. A team meeting has been planned for tomorrow. On the basis of the patient's current functional level you are concerned about her ability to return home.

What do you address at the meeting?

RESOLUTION

This patient underwent a major orthopedic surgical procedure and had chronic restrictive lung disease. These two factors compromised the patient's ability to supply oxygen to the tissues. The therapist checked the medical record and found that the patient's last hemoglobin level was 10 g/dL and the hematocrit was 28%. Both of these values were well below the normal values for women (14–18 g/dL and 33% to 43%, respectively). The therapist could not find any reference to the patient's blood gases or oximetry readings. At the team meeting the therapist recommended pulse oximetry monitoring. The following day blood gas readings were taken and yielded the following results:

	pH	pCO_2 (mmHg)	HCO_3 (Eq/L)	pO_2 (mmHg)	O_2 Saturation (%)
Resting	7.42	35	23	84	90

Pulse oximetry monitoring was performed at rest and during activities of daily living and exercise. After she ambulated 5 feet, the patient's oxygen saturation was 85%.

On the basis of the information obtained, the patient was provided with 2 L/min oxygen during all physical exertion. Oxygen was supplied when the patient performed transfers, self care, or attempted ambulation. The patient's diet was altered to enhance red blood cell replenishment, and iron supplements were provided.

The patient demonstrated an almost immediate increase in tolerance for exercise and activities of daily living. After 1 week, oxygen supplementation was decreased to 1 L/min. At the end of 2 weeks, oxygen supplementation was discontinued. Progress continued, and at the end of 3 weeks the patient was able to return home. Once home, the patient was provided with daily assistance by a home health aide and received home care physical therapy.

DISCUSSION

The combination of anemia and oxygen desaturation during activity was the cause of the patient's inability to progress. Desaturation is clinically significant when oxygen saturation readings drop below 90%. The combination of anemia and oxygen desaturation superimposed on pulmonary fibrosis (which by itself often contributes to decreased oxygen levels during exercise) can be extremely debilitating. The use of pulse oximetry, which is a noninvasive way of monitoring oxygen saturation, was invaluable in monitoring the increased physiologic demands placed on the patient.

The effects of general anesthesia (respiratory depression and decreased mucus transport) and immobility imposed by the patient's operation likely exacerbated the pulmonary disease and resulted in oxygen desaturation. The oxygen desaturation and anemia combined to decrease exercise tolerance. The good news was that these effects were temporary once they were identified and treated.

REFERENCES

Erannon FJ, Foley MW, Starr JA, Black MG: *Cardiopulmonary Rehabilitation: Basic Theory and Application,* second edition. Philadelphia: Davis, 1993.

Irwin S, Tecklin JS (ed): *Cardiopulmonary Physical Therapy,* second edition. St. Louis: Mosby Year Book, 1992.

Zadai CC (ed): *Pulmonary Management in Physical Therapy.* New York: Churchill Livingstone, 1992.

45

The Case of Cervical Tetraplegia

You are a senior physical therapist in a large urban rehabilitation center. One of your colleagues asks for your assistance regarding a 24-year-old man who was injured in a diving accident 4 weeks ago. The accident resulted in complete C-7 tetraplegia.

The patient's acute care was complicated by pneumonia that necessitated intubation and mechanical ventilation for 1 week. At present the patient is able to sit in a wheelchair 4 to 6 hours a day and requires no oxygen supplementation. The therapist treating the patient is becoming increasingly concerned because the patient is having difficulty participating in full-time rehabilitation. The patient reports shortness of breath and fatigue. The therapist indicates the patient remains very motivated to improve his condition. Your colleague is concerned that the patient will not achieve his rehabilitation goal of maximum functional independence.

How do you proceed?

RESOLUTION

With the multiple medical problems that patients such as this often present, it is possible to overlook various factors in the rehabilitation process. In this case, the cardiorespiratory problems that can occur in patients with tetraplegia likely affected all aspects of the rehabilitation program. The patient was suffering from restrictive pulmonary effects commonly associated with spinal cord injury and the loss of normal autonomic responses to changes of position during exercise.

The rehabilitation program was modified to include exercises to help improve respiratory muscle endurance and endurance of the remaining innervated muscles. The program also included techniques to prevent further immobilization of the chest wall and assisted cough techniques to maintain airway clearance. Within 4 days the patient was tolerating his treatment sessions with less fatigue. After 2 weeks the patient was able to tolerate rehabilitation of more than 4 hours of combined physical, occupational, and recreational therapy.

DISCUSSION

In addition to the range of motion, strength, and functional assessments performed on patients with spinal cord injuries, several other evaluations should be included. First, vital capacity should be measured while the patient is sitting and while he is supine. Next the patient's maximum inspiratory pressure, which is an indicator of respiratory muscle strength, should be measured with a negative pressure manometer. The patient's breathing pattern should be evaluated while the patient is supine to assess for paradoxic chest-wall motions commonly associated with tetraplegia. Other assessments include respiratory rate at rest and during exercise, palpation of the compliance of the rib cage, and the ability to exercise (e.g., monitor the ability to push a wheelchair for a distance over a period of time).

In this case, the therapist measured the patient's vital capacity as 1500 mL (approximately 35% of normal) and maximum inspiratory capacity as –45 cm H_2O (normal is –80 to –120 cm H_2O). The patient could push a wheelchair only 100 feet in 5 minutes before feeling shortness of breath and fatigue. Respiratory rate climbed to 30 breaths per minute. To address these problems, the patient performed a 10- to 15-minute a day inspiratory muscle training program using a spring-loaded inspiratory musculature training device. Also included in the program was distance wheelchair pushing, upper extremity ergometry, and guidelines for frequency and methods of proper coughing.

REFERENCES

Frownfelter DL (ed): *Chest Physical Therapy and Pulmonary Rehabilitation: An Interdisciplinary Approach*, second edition. St. Louis: Mosby Year Book, 1987.

Irwin S, Tecklin JS (eds): *Cardiopulmonary Physical Therapy*, second edition. St. Louis: Mosby Year Book, 1990.

Peat M (ed): *Current Physical Therapy*. Toronto: Decker, 1988.

46

The Case of the Patient with a Head Injury

Your patient is a 19-year-old woman who experienced a traumatic brain injury 6 months ago. She presents with mixed flaccid and mild spastic paralysis in all four extremities. Although the patient is able to ambulate short distances on a level surface using a quad cane, her right lower extremity exhibits foot drop during the swing phase of gait. There is also visible right genu recurvatum during the stance phase of gait. An orthosis was fabricated to prevent these gait deviations, but the weight of the orthosis was too heavy for the patient to lift. She wants to return to work at a flower shop but needs to walk to perform her duties.

What can you do to enable this patient to walk and control her gait deviations?

RESOLUTION

A portable, battery-operated functional electric stimulator (FES) was used as a substitute for the orthosis. A two-channel device with a heel switch control and the capability to activate channels alternately was required. The stimulator operated on the following stimulus parameters: balanced biphasic waveform, a phase duration of 300 microsec, frequency of 30 Hz, and an amplitude strong enough to stimulate fair to normal muscle contraction.

The electrodes used were as large as the area could support without stimulating contractions of surrounding muscles. Placement of the electrodes was parallel in orientation directly over target muscle fibers. Two electrodes from channel one were placed over the pretibial muscle group and the common peroneal nerve slightly below the head of the fibula. This electrode group was used to prevent foot drop during the swing phase of gait.

Two additional electrodes were placed over the hamstrings. Their purpose was to stimulate the hamstrings to prevent genu recurvatum during the stance phase of gait. The stimulator was set so channel one stimulated the pretibial group during swing phase (heel switch open) and channel two stimulated the hamstrings during stance phase (heel switch closed). The amplitude was adjusted to produce strong contractions and control unwanted motions.

DISCUSSION

The waveform characteristics presented have been well documented as being effective for FES. The rationale behind the stimulation of the pretibial group is to aid in the prevention of foot drop during the swing phase of gait. Although not a factor in this case, another possible cause of this gait deviation could be spasticity in the plantar flexor muscle group. If present, the muscle contraction induced in the pretibial group would need to be strong enough to overcome spasticity in the plantar flexors.

There is controversy among authorities whether stimulation of the gastrocnemius or the hamstrings can be most effective in preventing genu recurvatum during the stance phase of gait. The action of both muscles makes them likely candidates for FES orthotic substitution. The spasticity demonstrated by this patient dictated that stimulation of the hamstrings muscles would be effective in preventing the observed gait deviations.

REFERENCES

Alon G: High voltage stimulation: effects of electrode size on basic excitatory responses. Phys Ther 1985;65:890–895.

Baker LL, Parker K, Sanderson D: Neuromuscular electrical stimulation for the head-injured patient. Phys Ther 1983;63:1967–1974.

Bogatij U, Gros N, Malezic M, et al: Restoration of gait during two to three weeks of therapy with multichannel electrical stimulation. Phys Ther 1989;69:319–327.

Brooks MS, Smith EM, Currier DP: Effect of longitudinal versus transverse electrode placement on torque production by the quadriceps femoris muscle during neuromuscular stimulation. J Orthop Phys Ther 1990;11:530–534.

Gersh M (ed): *Electrotherapy in Rehabilitation*. Philadelphia: Davis, 1992.

Nelson RM, Currier DP (eds): *Clinical Electrotherapy*, second edition. Norwalk: Appleton & Lange, 1991.

47

The Case of Hip Bursitis

Your patient is a 72-year-old woman who returned home yesterday after 2 weeks in a rehabilitation center following left total hip replacement. The operation went well, and the patient was able to complete a comprehensive rehabilitation program. She had progressed to unassisted ambulation, bearing weight as tolerated, with a quad cane. Three days before the patient left the rehabilitation center, however, the staff physiatrist diagnosed right hip bursitis. The physician attributed the bursitis to overactivity.

You evaluate the patient and find she needs a walker to ambulate and reports right buttock pain. While ambulating the patient positions the right lower extremity in slight external rotation and lands flat-footed on the left foot. She prematurely and quickly swings the right leg forward during the left leg stance phase. The patient denies any pain in the left leg and says the problem is constant right buttock pain. With a sense of frustration she abruptly states, "I don't think I'll ever get rid of this pain."

How do you proceed?

RESOLUTION

This case demonstrates the complex nature of pain and why a thorough evaluation is always indicated. With additional questioning the therapist determined that the initial "bursitis" pain was not at all localized but radiated down the leg and into the toes. The location of the reported pain was in the right midgluteal area and increased with palpation.

While performing a manual muscle test the therapist observed that resisted lateral right hip rotation was painful and that overpressure at end range of medial rotation increased the pain. Palpation over the piriformis muscle also reproduced the pain. Flexibility testing showed a small loss of mobility in the right hip but a marked loss in the left. The patient was unable to actively extend the left hip beyond 30 degrees of flexion.

To address the problems presented, the therapist instituted a gentle program of stretching of the anterior musculature of both lower extremities. The program also emphasized stretching the right hip external rotators. After 2 days the patient reported an absence of pain, and 15 days later all gait deviations had been eliminated. The patient advanced from a quad to a straight cane and was discharged from home physical therapy.

DISCUSSION

The patient in this case was progressing normally after left total hip replacement. The pain in the uninvolved lower extremity was attributed to overexertion. Although it is pos-sible the patient may have overexerted herself, other factors, including lack of flexibility in both lower extremities, should have been considered. The nature of the pain (radiating down the entire extremity) indicated that a diagnosis of bursitis was unlikely. Spasm of the piriformis muscle can irritate the sciatic nerve, causing pain along the entire sciatic distribution. Even as a spasm resolves, pain may continue in the immediate area for some time.

The flexibility limitations observed in this patient were related to the fact that the patient performed postoperative hip mobility exercises while standing in parallel bars. The patient did not have accurate visual cues and was performing the exercises while maintaining a flexed trunk. To compensate for markedly reduced left hip extension during gait, the patient externally rotated her right lower extremity and increased the right swing speed. Those compensations apparently stressed the external rotators of the right hip, resulting in inflammation and spasm. After several days of careful stretching, the patient regained lost flexibility, relieved the stressed musculature, and resumed a normal gait pattern.

REFERENCES

Bonder BR, Wagner MB (eds): *Functional Performance in Older Adults*. Philadelphia: Davis, 1994.

Guccione AA (ed): *Geriatric Physical Therapy*. St. Louis: Mosby Year Book, 1993.

Rich BSE, McKeag D: When sciatica is not disk disease: detecting piriformis syndrome in active patients. Phys Sports Med 1992;20:104–108,111,115.

48

The Case of
Achilles Tendon Pain

Your colleague requests assistance with a 38-year-old woman who has been referred to the facility because of bilateral Achilles tendon pain. The patient indicates she has been an avid walker for many years, having progressed to 5 miles per day. Recently, however, she has begun to experience an insidious onset of bilateral Achilles pain, which has become so debilitating that normal ambulation is painful. During the initial evaluation it was found that the Achilles tendons and gastrocnemius and soleus muscles of both legs were tender to touch. In fact, a node was forming at the right mid-Achilles tendon.

To date treatment has consisted of phonophoresis, transverse friction massage, deep massage to both gastrocnemius and soleus muscle groups, and instruction for standing gastrocnemius muscle stretching. After treatment, a 58°F whirlpool is used for 15 minutes, and Achilles straps are applied. After 2 weeks of treatment the patient demonstrates only moderate progress. Pain continues to be clinically significant despite only minimal ambulation.

How do you recommend treatment proceed?

RESOLUTION

Upon further evaluation, the therapist found that the patient had an apparent leg length discrepancy (right longer than left), pelvic asymmetry with the right anterior superior iliac spine inferior to the left, and a positive standing Thomas test. There was pain with palpation of the left posterior superior iliac spine and surrounding muscles and palpable paravertebral muscle spasm (left greater than right). All objective findings were consistent with a posterior rotation of the left sacroiliac joint. Evidence indicated a biomechanical cause had led to a gait deviation and a secondary onset of bilateral Achilles tendinitis.

Treatment was modified to include instructing the patient in a self-mobilization technique to correct the sacroiliac joint alignment. (If this form of treatment had not been successful, the therapist would have had to perform passive joint mobilization.) As a result, the patient began to experience pain-free ambulation and a progressive decrease in bilateral Achilles tendon symptoms. The patient continued to perform flexibility exercises and self-mobilization before her daily walks.

DISCUSSION

Sacroiliac joint mobilization and treatment is a clinical skill understood and applied by many practitioners. The nature of dysfunction is often one of long-term hypermobility of the joint (and hypomobility of related joints), which if left untreated, results in considerable discomfort. If self-mobilization techniques are consistently and successfully applied, an essentially pain-free condition may be maintained.

REFERENCES

Maitland GD: *Vertebral Manipulation*, fifth edition. Boston: Butterworth-Heinemann, 1986.

Mayer TG, Mooney V, Gatchel RJ: *Contemporary Conservative Care for Painful Spinal Disorders*. Malvern: Lea & Febiger, 1991.

Wadsworth CT: *Manual Examination and Treatment of the Spine and Extremities*. Baltimore: Williams & Wilkins, 1988.

Afterword

As the nature and complexity of health care continue to evolve, the profession of physical therapy will be called upon to assume greater responsibility in providing patient care services. For the physical therapist, the key to attaining and applying high-level skills on a regular basis is the acquisition of knowledge. Increasingly the expectation is that we, as professionals, be able to determine the cause of complex patient care problems and solve them before an adverse result occurs. To do this requires an ability to recognize how quickly a problem can arise and what must be done to prevent undesirable consequences.

The knowledge needed to perform at a high skill level comes only with dedication. To grow in professional knowledge you must define your clinical expectations and maintain constant effort toward achieving high performance standards. People who become leaders in the profession of physical therapy set realistic goals and reach them. They learn to overcome setbacks that occur and structure conditions for success. Most important, physical therapists who excel at what they do, and report experiencing high professional rewards, are those who become immersed in their activities. In other words, they sustain involvement.

To increase your professional skills and abilities, seek opportunities to watch others knowledgeable in a clinical area. Try to volunteer for patient care treatment assignments that allow you to work with other therapists who excel at what they do. Once you learn to recognize the qualities that constitute excellence in patient care, you begin to acquire the knowledge base of experience.

As you practice your new professional skills and abilities, ask others to provide you with constructive feedback regarding performance. Hearing constructive feedback from those we respect helps enhance the acquisition of clinical competence. Above all, try to work in an environment where opportunities for learning abound and where there is a team concept in listening to, addressing, and solving complex patient care problems.

Index

compression stockings, 52, 72
congenital defects
    delayed ambulation, 35–36
    low-muscle-tone infant, 35–36, 79–80
congestive heart failure, 4
    identifying, 71–72, 83–84
COPD. *See* chronic obstructive pulmonary
    disease

degenerative disk disease, cervical, 41–42
denervation, muscles. *See* muscle
    denervation
developmental delay, 79
diabetic patient, abrasion from prosthesis,
    33–34
disk problems, cervical, 41–42
dizziness
    orthostatic hypotension, 71–72
    vertebral artery test, 11–12
dragging, leg, 13–14
drug therapy
    age of medication, 15–16
    coordination with physical therapy, 69–70
    over-the-counter medicines, 84
    unsuccessful, 4
dyspnea
    amyotrophic lateral sclerosis, 43–44
    congestive heart failure, 72, 83–84
    elderly patient, 71–72
    emphysema patient, 73–74

ear problems, elderly, 45–46
edema
    ankle, postsurgical, 67
    compression stockings, 51–52
    congestive heart failure, 3–4, 71–72
    peripheral, 51–52, 71–72
elbow, painful, 29–30
elderly patients
    congestive heart failure, 71–72, 83–84
    ear problems, 45–46
    shortness of breath, 71–72
    visual changes, 43–44
    weak spell, 83–84
electrical stimulation
    Bell's palsy, 77
    diagnostic, 28
    functional electrical stimulator, 92
    gait correction, 92
    Wallerian degeneration, 78
emphysema patient, dyspnea, 73–74

exercise
    breathing exercises, 43–44, 73–74, 89–90
    soft tissue stretching, 65
    too aggressive, 60
exercise tolerance
    cardiomyopathy, 69–70
    chronic obstructive pulmonary disease,
        19–20
    emphysema patient, 73–74
    pulmonary fibrosis, 87–88
    tetraplegia, cervical, 89–90
eye problems, 13–14, 31–32

face, Bell's palsy, 77–78
family education, oxygen administration, 20
fatigue, muscular dystrophy symptom, 13–14
fever, orthopedic patient, 7–8
flexibility, testing, 23, 57, 94
foot
    pain, 22, 67–68
    splinter discovered, 25–26
foot drop, 91–92
fracture
    cast, pain and numbness, 5–6
    muscle denervation, 27–28
    painful gait, 21–22
    scapular, 49–50
functional electrical stimulator (FES), head
    injury, 91–92

gait
    Achilles tendon pain, 95–96
    brain injury, 91–92
    dragging leg, 13–14
    elderly patients, 31–32, 45–46
    foot drop, 91–92
    genu recurvatum, 91–92
    handicapped child, 35–36
    hip replacement, 17–18, 93–94
    muscular dystrophy, 13–14
    painful, following fracture, 21–22
    pronation, 58
    prosthesis, 33–34
    knee weakness following replacement,
        23–24
general conditioning, unsuccessful, 13–14
genu recurvatum, 91–92

headaches, cervical and TMJ dysfunction,
    55–56

shoulder pain
    cervical and TMJ dysfunction, 56
    in stroke victim, 49–50
    scapular fracture, 49–50
    torticollis, 81–82
soft-tissue stretching, cerebral palsy, 65–66
spinal cord, tumor, 48
spinal pain
    cervical, 41–42
    wheelchair removal from car causing,
        37–38
spine
    injury, respiratory effects, 90
    muscular atrophy, 63–64
    scoliosis, 63–64
splinter wound, recognizing, 25
spring test, 39
stress loading, reflex sympathetic dystrophy,
    61–62
stroke. *See* cerebral vascular accident
swelling, thrombophlebitis, 3–4
sympathetic dystrophy, arm, 61–62
syncope, compression stockings, 52
synovial joints, postsurgical edema, 67

temporomandibular joint dysfunction
    (TMJ), 56
tendon lengthening, 35–36
tendon, torn. *See* torn tendon
terrible triad, 7
TENS unit, 62
tetraplegia, cervical, 89–90
thrombophlebitis, 4
tibia
    compartment syndrome, 53–54
    pain in healed fracture, 21
    plateau fracture, 5–6
tibia-fibula fracture
    muscle denervation, 27–28
    painful gait following, 21–22
torn tendon
    biceps, 30
    quadriceps, 23–24

torticollis, 81–82
traction, neck pain, 12, 81–82
transfers, 17, 43, 45, 65, 69, 71, 75, 87
trapezius muscle, spasm, 11–12, 82
tumor, spinal cord, 47–48
two-joint muscles, 29

ulcer, ankle, wound treatment, 85–86
urinary tract infection, symptoms,
    39–40

vertebral artery test, 12
visual acuity
    as diagnostic symptom, 13–14
    glare in the elderly, 31–32

walker, emphysema patient, 74
Wallerian degeneration, 78
weakness due to compression following
    joint replacement, 47
weightbearing, postsurgical return to,
    67–68
wet-to-dry dressings, 86
wheelchair
    difficulty transfering, 65
    removal from car causing spinal pain,
        37–38
whiplash injury, 11–12
whirlpool. *See* hydrotherapy
work activities modification, 41
work injury. *See* industrial injury
wound debridement
    bleeding, 1–2
    HIV-positive patient, 9–10
    hydrotherapy, 25–26
    splinter discovered, 25–26
wound treatment, alginate dressings,
    86

x-ray, shortcomings, 25–26